Paper Doctors
(First published 1977)

Vernon Coleman

Vernon Coleman: What the papers say:

'Vernon Coleman writes as a general practitioner who has become disquieted by the all-pervasive influence of the pharmaceutical industry in modern medicine...He describes, with a wealth of illustrations, the phenomena of modern iatrogenesis; but he is also concerned about the wider harm which can result from doctors' and patients' preoccupation with medication instead of with the prevention of disease. He demonstrates, all the more effectively because he writes in a sober, matter-of-fact style, the immense influence exercised by the drug industry on doctors' prescribing habits...He writes as a family doctor who is keenly aware of the social dimensions of medical practice. He ends his book with practical suggestions as to how medical care – in the developing countries as well as in the West – can best be freed from this unhealthy pharmaceutical predominance.' – G.M.Carstairs, The Times Literary Supplement (1975)

'What he says of the present is true: and it is the great merit of the book that he says it from the viewpoint of a practising general practitioner, who sees from the inside what is going on, and is appalled by the consequences to the profession, and to the public.' – Brian Inglis, Punch (1975)

'Dr Coleman writes with more sense than bias. Required reading for any Minister of Health' – Daily Express

'I hope this book becomes a bestseller among doctors, nurses and the wider public...' – Nursing Times

'Dr Coleman's well-coordinated book could not be more timely.' – Yorkshire Post

'Few would disagree with Dr Coleman that more should be done about prevention.' – The Lancet

'This short but very readable book has a message that is timely. Vernon Coleman's point is that much of the medical research into which money and expertise are poured is useless. At the same time, remedial conditions of mind and body which cause the most distress are largely neglected. This is true.' – Daily Telegraph

'If you believe Dr Vernon Coleman, the main beneficiaries of the hundred million pounds worth of research done in this country each year are certainly not the patients. The research benefits mostly the medical place seekers, who use their academic investigations as rungs on the promotional ladder, or drug companies with an eye for the latest market opening…The future may hold bionic superman but all a nation's physic cannot significantly change the basic mortality statistics except sometimes, to make them worse.' – The Guardian

'Dr Coleman's well-coordinated book could not be more timely.' – Yorkshire Post

'The Medicine Men is well worth reading' – Times Educational Supplement

'Dr Vernon Coleman…is not a mine of information – he is a fountain. It pours out of him, mixed with opinions which have an attractive common sense ring about them.' – Coventry Evening Telegraph

'The Medicine Men' by Dr Vernon Coleman, was the subject of a 14 minute 'commercial' on the BBC's Nationwide television programme recently. Industry doctors and general practitioners come in for a severe drubbing: two down and several more to go because the targets for Dr Coleman's pen are many, varied and, to say the least, surprising. Take the physicians who carry out clinical trials: many of those, claims the author, have sold themselves to the industry and agreed to do research for rewards of one kind or another, whether that reward be a trip abroad, a piece of equipment, a few dinners, a series of published papers or simply money.' – The Pharmaceutical Journal

'When the children have finished playing the games on your Sinclair or Commodore Vic 20 computer, you can turn it to more practical purposes. For what is probably Britain's first home doctor programme for computers is now available. Dr Vernon Coleman, one of the country's leading medical authors, has prepared the text for a remarkable series of six cassettes called The Home Doctor Series. Dr Coleman, author of the new book 'Bodypower'…has turned his attention to computers.' – The Times 1983

'By the year 2020 there will be a holocaust, not caused by a plutonium plume but by greed, medical ambition and political opportunism. This is the latest vision of Vernon Coleman, an articulate and prolific medical author…this disturbing book detects diseases in the whole way we deliver health care.' – Sunday Times (1988)

`…the issues explores he explores are central to the health of the nation.' – Nursing Times

'It is not necessary to accept his conclusion to be able to savour his decidedly trenchant comments on today's medicine…a book to stimulate and to make one argue.' – British Medical Journal

``As a writer of medical bestsellers, Dr Vernon Coleman's aim is to shock us out of our complacency…it's impossible not to be impressed by some of his arguments.' – Western Daily Press

`Controversial and devastating' – Publishing News

`Dr Coleman produces mountains of evidence to justify his outrageous claims.' – Edinburgh Evening News

`Dr Coleman lays about him with an uncompromising verbal scalpel, dipped in vitriol, against all sorts of sacred medical cows.' – Exeter Express and Echo

'Vernon Coleman writes brilliant books.' – The Good Book Guide

'No thinking person can ignore him. This is why he has been for over 20 years one of the world's leading advocates on human and animal rights in relation to health. Long may it continue.' – The Ecologist

'The calmest voice of reason comes from Dr Vernon Coleman.' – The Observer

'A godsend.' – Daily Telegraph

`Dr Vernon Coleman has justifiably acquired a reputation for being controversial, iconoclastic and influential.' – General Practitioner

'Superstar.' – Independent on Sunday

'Brilliant!' – The People

'Compulsive reading.' – The Guardian

'His message is important.' – The Economist

'He's the Lone Ranger, Robin Hood and the Equalizer rolled into one.' – Glasgow Evening Times

'The man is a national treasure.' – What Doctors Don't Tell You

'His advice is optimistic and enthusiastic.' – British Medical Journal

'Revered guru of medicine.' – Nursing Times

'Gentle, kind and caring' – Western Daily Press

'His trademark is that he doesn't mince words. Far funnier than the usual tone of soupy piety you get from his colleagues.' – The Guardian

Books by Vernon Coleman include:

Medical
The Medicine Men
Paper Doctors
Everything You Want To Know About Ageing
The Home Pharmacy
Aspirin or Ambulance
Face Values
Stress and Your Stomach
A Guide to Child Health
Guilt
The Good Medicine Guide
An A to Z of Women's Problems
Bodypower
Bodysense
Taking Care of Your Skin
Life without Tranquillisers
High Blood Pressure
Diabetes
Arthritis
Eczema and Dermatitis
The Story of Medicine
Natural Pain Control
Mindpower
Addicts and Addictions
Dr Vernon Coleman's Guide to Alternative Medicine
Stress Management Techniques
Overcoming Stress
The Health Scandal
The 20 Minute Health Check
Sex for Everyone
Mind over Body
Eat Green Lose Weight
Why Doctors Do More Harm Than Good
The Drugs Myth

Complete Guide to Sex
How to Conquer Backache
How to Conquer Pain
Betrayal of Trust
Know Your Drugs
Food for Thought
The Traditional Home Doctor
Relief from IBS
The Parent's Handbook
Men in Bras, Panties and Dresses
Power over Cancer
How to Conquer Arthritis
How to Stop Your Doctor Killing You
Superbody
Stomach Problems – Relief at Last
How to Overcome Guilt
How to Live Longer
Coleman's Laws
Millions of Alzheimer Patients Have Been Misdiagnosed
Climbing Trees at 112
Is Your Health Written in the Stars?
The Kick-Ass A–Z for over 60s
Briefs Encounter
The Benzos Story
Dementia Myth
Waiting

Psychology/Sociology
Stress Control
How to Overcome Toxic Stress
Know Yourself (1988)
Stress and Relaxation
People Watching
Spiritpower
Toxic Stress
I Hope Your Penis Shrivels Up
Oral Sex: Bad Taste and Hard To Swallow
Other People's Problems

The 100 Sexiest, Craziest, Most Outrageous Agony Column
Questions (and Answers) Of All Time
How to Relax and Overcome Stress
Too Sexy To Print
Psychiatry
Are You Living With a Psychopath?

Politics and General
England Our England
Rogue Nation
Confronting the Global Bully
Saving England
Why Everything Is Going To Get Worse Before It Gets Better
The Truth They Won't Tell You...About The EU
Living In a Fascist Country
How to Protect & Preserve Your Freedom, Identity & Privacy
Oil Apocalypse
Gordon is a Moron
The OFPIS File
What Happens Next?
Bloodless Revolution
2020
Stuffed
The Shocking History of the EU
Coming Apocalypse
Covid-19: The Greatest Hoax in History
Old Man in a Chair
Endgame
Proof that Masks do more Harm than Good
Covid-19: The Fraud Continues
Covid-19: Exposing the Lies
Social Credit: Nightmare on Your Street
NHS: What's wrong and how to put it right
They want your money and your life.

Diaries and Autobiographies
Diary of a Disgruntled Man
Just another Bloody Year

Bugger off and Leave Me Alone
Return of the Disgruntled Man
Life on the Edge
The Game's Afoot
Tickety Tonk
Memories 1
Memories 2
My Favourite Books

Animals
Why Animal Experiments Must Stop
Fighting For Animals
Alice and Other Friends
Animal Rights – Human Wrongs
Animal Experiments – Simple Truths

General Non Fiction
How to Publish Your Own Book
How to Make Money While Watching TV
Strange but True
Daily Inspirations
Why Is Public Hair Curly
People Push Bottles Up Peaceniks
Secrets of Paris
Moneypower
101 Things I Have Learned
100 Greatest Englishmen and Englishwomen
Cheese Rolling, Shin Kicking and Ugly Tattoos
One Thing after Another

Novels (General)
Mrs Caldicot's Cabbage War
Mrs Caldicot's Knickerbocker Glory
Mrs Caldicot's Oyster Parade
Mrs Caldicot's Turkish Delight
Deadline
Second Chance
Tunnel

Mr Henry Mulligan
The Truth Kills
Revolt
My Secret Years with Elvis
Balancing the Books
Doctor in Paris
Stories with a Twist in the Tale (short stories)
Dr Bullock's Annals

The Young Country Doctor Series
Bilbury Chronicles
Bilbury Grange
Bilbury Revels
Bilbury Country
Bilbury Village
Bilbury Pie (short stories)
Bilbury Pudding (short stories)
Bilbury Tonic
Bilbury Relish
Bilbury Mixture
Bilbury Delights
Bilbury Joys
Bilbury Tales
Bilbury Days
Bilbury Memories

Novels (Sport)
Thomas Winsden's Cricketing Almanack
Diary of a Cricket Lover
The Village Cricket Tour
The Man Who Inherited a Golf Course
Around the Wicket
Too Many Clubs and Not Enough Balls

Cat books
Alice's Diary
Alice's Adventures
We Love Cats

Cats Own Annual
The Secret Lives of Cats
Cat Basket
The Cataholics' Handbook
Cat Fables
Cat Tales
Catoons from Catland

As Edward Vernon
Practice Makes Perfect
Practise What You Preach
Getting Into Practice
Aphrodisiacs – An Owner's Manual
The Complete Guide to Life

Written with Donna Antoinette Coleman
How to Conquer Health Problems between Ages 50 & 120
Health Secrets Doctors Share With Their Families
Animal Miscellany
England's Glory
Wisdom of Animals

Dedication

This edition is dedicated to Antoinette – my wife, my love, my dearest friend.
With all my love.
Always and All Ways

Contents

Introduction to 2023 Edition

I started work on *Paper Doctors* in 1975 immediately after the
publication of *The Medicine Men* and continued to work on it in
1976. Maurice Temple-Smith, who had published *The Medicine Men*
also published *Paper Doctors* and I think it was Maurice who
thought up the title. He was a wonderful, old-fashioned publisher
who worked in offices opposite the British Museum. I seem to
remember that his older authors had no little difficulty climbing the
narrow, steep, slightly rickety staircase. As with all small publishers
in those days there were stacks of books piled everywhere. M T-S
was kind and patient and I was sad when he retired. While I was
researching *The Medicine Men* (which described in depth the
relationship between the medical profession and the pharmaceutical
industry) I had discovered much about medical research which had
appalled me and so this book was inevitable. Re-reading *Paper
Doctors* recently I realised just how relevant the book still is and I
was saddened to discover that only one copy of the book still existed
– in America. I bought that copy through Abe Books (for $250 plus
$25 postage), had it scanned and published it myself in the belief
that it will be of interest to readers today, but also in the knowledge
that it's now a fairly esoteric title and I'll probably not sell enough
copies to cover the cost of the book and the scanning. Some of the
writing in the book now seems rather clumsy (it would be strange if
it did not since I was in my 20s when I wrote it and I hope I've
learned a little since then) but I have resisted the temptation to make
any changes. I've republished the book as it was when it first came
out. I dug out the review file and I'm pleased to see that the
reviewers were very kind. The *Daily Express* said the book was
'required reading for any Minister of Health'. The *Daily Telegraph*
described the book as very readable and having a timely message.
The Guardian spotted my conclusion that 'the main beneficiaries of
the hundred million pounds worth of medical research done in this
country each year are certainly not the patients'. *The Lancet* said that
'Few would disagree with Dr Coleman'. The *Nursing Times*
reviewer said: 'I hope this book becomes a bestseller among doctors,

nurses and the wider public who, after all, have to pay for the research'. I couldn't find a bad review in my file, though I suppose it is possible that any bad reviews might have been discarded decades ago, or never retained. Surprisingly, even *Chemist and Druggist* had kind things to say about *Paper Doctors*.

Vernon Coleman, January 2023

No table of contents entries found.

Preface

In the last two or three years a number of authors have fiercely attacked the medical profession as being largely unnecessary. Some have argued that doctors cause more illness than they cure. I do not agree that we could manage better without doctors but I do believe that doctors at present have got their priorities wrong. Far too much emphasis is laid on the collection of new information and too little on the use of information already available. Medicine is an industry of which formal medical research is an integral part. Medical researchers have an extraordinary amount of influence within the medical profession and consume vast amounts of time and money whilst their colleagues working in the field of preventive medicine receive little of either. Too many medical researchers are doing work of doubtful value which could best be justified as a medical luxury only suitable for a world in which there was little illness and little suffering. At worst, medical research programmes are often dangerous and destructive.

I am not alone in my belief that medical research is largely irrelevant in our modern world. In the first two chapters of this book I give the main reasons why I and many others in the medical profession feel that medical research programmes should be curtailed and the money and effort used elsewhere. In Chapters 3 to 11 I have tried to illustrate the arguments outlined in the first two chapters and to provide the facts to support my thesis.

The final chapters of the book describe how I think we should be using our medical resources. Since a totally destructive book would leave a void, I have tried to explain in some detail why I think there are more important areas for support than traditional medical research programmes

1. Historical Introduction

Traditionally doctors have believed that improvements in health will automatically follow if we acquire a greater under-standing of the structure and function, and hence the diseased structure and malfunction, of the human body. It is not difficult to show that modern medical practice developed during the last two centuries and that during the same interval life expectation increased at a faster rate than ever before.

The reliable identification of disease began in the nineteenth century, as did the first accurate understanding of disease processes. The ancient physicians had always blamed the development of disease on the defective mixing of the 'humours', in the body but in 1761 an Italian called Giovanni Battista Morgagni published a book entitled *On the Seats and Causes of Diseases* based on a great number of post mortems in which he showed convincingly that different diseases involve different organs. Forty years later a Frenchman, Marie Francois Xavier Bichat, showed that organs are made up of many different kinds of tissue and that different tissues are responsible for different disease processes.

In 1833 a German, Johannes Muller, published the first volume of his *Handbook of Human Physiology* which led the move away from philosophical medicine towards a more scientific approach. The final and perhaps most important step in the creation of the basis of modern medical thought was taken in 1855 by another German, Rudolf Virchow, who used microscopes to study cells and who introduced the idea of 'cellular pathology'. His book called *Cellular Pathology* as based upon *Physiological and Pathological History* was published in 1858 and many historians believe that it marked the beginning of modern medicine.

The fight against infection was also fought with great enthusiasm in the nineteenth century. Jan Ignaz Semmelweis, an assistant in the Obstetrics Unit in Vienna believed that puerperal fever, an infection which affects women who have just given birth, was caused by a poison of some sort from dead bodies. He was scorned and his theories were rejected at first but later in the same century he was proved right. Robert Koch discovered the tubercle bacillus in. 1882 and in 1883 found the organism which cause cholera. In the 1860s Pasteur developed his theory of the cause of infectious diseases. It was in 1865 that Joseph Lister, the British surgeon, developed the antisepsis principle which helped to save patients on the operating table. Before Lister came along surgeons used to wear their oldest and dirtiest clothes in the operating theatre and their instruments were rarely if ever rinsed.

The basis of modern anaesthesia was developed in the nineteenth century. Horace Wells, an American dentist, introduced the use of nitrous oxide (laughing gas) in 1844; another American, William Thomas Green Morton, first used ether in 1846, and a Scottish doctor, Sir James Young Simpson, introduced chloroform as a general anaesthetic in 1847. He complained that '... the man who lies on the operating table in one of our hospitals runs a greater risk of dying than did the British soldier on the Battlefield of Waterloo.'

The compound microscope, which enabled Virchow to study cells and Pasteur to study micro-organisms associated with different diseases, was developed during the nineteenth century, and in 1895, at the end of this scientifically magnificent century, Roentgen, who at the time was engaged in basic physics research, discovered X-rays and, almost accidentally, made the greatest single contribution to diagnostic medicine. Like a good many of the inventions later to prove so vital to doctors, the X-ray machine was developed by someone who had no interest at all in medical practice or medical research.

No one could deny that the nineteenth century saw the introduction of many of the ideas and techniques which are so important to the modern medical practitioner. Through the efforts of researchers medical men had learnt a great deal about the function and structure of the human body. Never before had a single century seen a greater increase in the amount of medical knowledge made available. It is doubtful whether a similar 'information explosion' will ever occur again.

During that same century when Virchow, Pasteur and Koch were making their great. discoveries, the expectation of life undeniably improved quite dramatically. A baby born two centuries ago would on average live only to the age of 25 years. By the end of the nineteenth century, however, the new-born baby had a far better chance of reaching his biblically allotted three score years and ten. The one-year-old male would, in 1901, stand an average chance of living to the age of 55; the 45-year-old male could expect another 23 years of life. During no other century had life expectation improved so dramatically.

It would be surprising if some observers had not concluded that this improvement was related directly to the accumulation of information. However, it is clear, in retrospect, that such a conclusion would be a mistake. The fact is that it was the increase in the supply of good food, the increase in the supply of pure water and the improvement in the quality of available housing which had the greatest effect. Cholera, for example, one of the biggest 'killers' of the nineteenth century, was brought under control by hygienic measures years before Koch discovered the existence of the cholera vibrio, and the decline in the incidence of tuberculosis was due not to the discovery of the tubercle bacillus but to improved nutritional standards.

According to Thomas McKeown and C.F. Lowe, authors of *An introduction to Social Medicine* and respectively Professor of Social Medicine at the University of Birmingham and Professor of Social and Occupational Medicine at the Welsh National School of Medicine, '... it seems right to conclude that in descending order of importance the main influences responsible for the decline in mortality – our best index of improved health – since deaths were first registered in 1838 have been: a rising standard of living, hygienic measures and specific preventive and curative medicine.' A WHO publication entitled *Life Expectancy in the Year 2000* adds stable government, progress in road building and better education to this list.

From the middle of the nineteenth century improvements in food available, in the quality of water supplies, in sanitation, in living accommodation and other environmental factors were largely responsible for the fact that typhoid, scarlet fever, dysentery and infective diarrhoeas were brought under some sort of control. These diseases were important killers at that time and their environmental control led to a direct drop in mortality rates. The many technically important discoveries of the nineteenth century were of far more importance to the academic than to the busy practitioner struggling with the practical problems of how to treat disease. Vaccination against smallpox was one of the very few medical measures to have any real effect in the nineteenth century and smallpox was of relatively small importance in statistical terms.

During the twentieth century medical intervention did play a much greater part in the improvement of life expectation. By far the greatest contribution to medical care came from the researchers developing drugs. At the end of the nineteenth century the pharmaceutical industry was still in its infancy (the first aspirin tablet was made in 1899) but during the next three or four decades great advances (many of them accidental) were made in the development of drugs. The discovery of the hormone insulin by Banting, Best and Murphy in 1922 brought about a revolution in the treatment of diabetics. The development of potent diuretics and drugs to control hypertension meant that patients with cardiovascular disorders could be treated. In 1914 Wenckebach discovered the usefulness of quinidine for patients suffering from arrhythmias of the heart. And there were, of course, tremendous advances in the development of drugs with which to control infectious diseases. The development of the sulphonamides, the penicillin and so on meant that those infectious diseases which still remained were no longer the threat that they had been.

The resultant more effective treatment of infectious diseases helped to ensure that life expectancy rose from fifty years at the beginning of the century to about seventy years today. There were over 40,000 deaths from tuberculosis in England and Wales in 1925 but only about 1,500 in 1970. There were over 6,000 deaths from whooping cough in 1925 but only 15 in 1970. More than 5,000 people died from measles in 1925 but by 1970 the annual mortality rate had dropped below 50. The mortality from gastro-intestinal infections has dropped by 80 per cent in the United Kingdom since 1930 and the number of deaths from chest infections has dropped by 70 per cent in the same period.

Interestingly, the improvement in life expectancy which we have enjoyed in this century has been largely due to the fact that there has been a dramatic decrease in the number of children dying. In 1900 about 150 children in every 1000 born in England and Wales died within one year. By 1950 this figure was down to 30.

Adults, however, have benefited far less from the pharmaceutical revolution. If we consider their life expectancy, we find that it has hardly changed in the last three-quarters of a century. The 45-year-old male could expect another 23 years in 1901 and only another 25 years in 1971. The improvement in standards of nutrition and in living standards generally had very much affected the life expectation of the middle-aged man in the second half of the nineteenth century; in the first half of the twentieth Century it was the survival rate of infants which was most improved.

There have, of course, been a number of discoveries outside the drug field in the twentieth century. The most important of these was probably that of a young Viennese scientist, Karl Landsteiner, who in 1901 found that blood transfusion between human beings was possible if the patient received blood from a donor with the same group. Other advances have often been concerned with small numbers of patients suffering from specific, well-defined disease processes. There have, for example, been advances in the treatment of many congenital disorders and there have been improvements and additions to the range of diagnostic equipment available. The twentieth century has seen the introduction of the artificial heart valve, the artificial kidney, the cardiac catheter, the potassium counting machine, ultrasound and so on. All of these have taken a great deal of effort and money but none have made any great contribution to general improvement in the quality of life this century.

Improvements in life expectation in the twentieth century have been largely due to the better living conditions, better preventive medicine techniques, improved surgical techniques and greater availability of drug therapy, which were all made possible by the efforts and successes of men and women who worked before most of us were born. It seems clear, therefore, that, with the single important exception of drugs for the treatment of infectious diseases, medical research has had surprisingly little effect on life expectation. Improvement in human health in the late nineteenth and early twentieth centuries has been largely due to changes in the environment and modifications in human behaviour.

What, then, have been the effects of medical research on life expectation during the first two decades of the second half of the twentieth century? After all, there has been an enormous increase in the amount of money and effort poured into medical research and never before have there been so many people directly involved in health care programmes.

Astonishingly, there has been almost no improvement in life expectation for young or for old. A recent World Health Organisation study has shown, in fact, that in a number of industrial countries the life expectancy of people over the age of sixty has actually started to fall. In the United States, where expenditure on health care is enormous, life expectancy for men and women of all ages is falling. Infant mortality rates are rising in many developed countries. Even the quality of life does not seem to have improved: about one third of all young Americans called up for the Vietnam draft, were rejected for medical or psychiatric reasons.

The facts that hospitals are continuing to grow, that hospital waiting lists are increasing all the time, that the amount of sick leave taken by working men and women seems to rise each year, that mental illnesses are getting commoner every time statistics are brought up to date, that the incidence of heart disease seems to be on the increase, that there is a massive increase in the amount of pollutant-inspired illness, that 80 per cent of modern cancers are thought to be caused by chemicals of one sort or another, and that the number of health professionals needed to cope with all the sick is increasing rapidly, seem to suggest that medical research has had relatively little effect on the morbidity rates or upon the quality of life at any time. In the last century. In addition, there is evidence that medical research has actually detracted from the quality of life, causing ethical problems and using funds which could be better used on projects more likely to contribute to it. Since the arguments supporting continued expenditure of large sums on medical research must depend primarily on the success of medical researchers in contributing to an improvement in the quantity of life we all enjoy, and secondarily on their success in contributing to its quality, it is difficult to see how one can argue in favour of sustaining our current high levels of expenditure on medical research.

Indeed, there is not only evidence for the uselessness of much medical research: there are also sound indications that many developed countries have reached a point of over-medication which is harmful to health. In developed countries, if a patient has two conditions – two diseases – there is a very good chance indeed that one of those diseases was caused by the treatment for the other.

Writing in the *Journal of Human Resources*, an American researcher, Charles T. Stewart, has shown that life expectation is approximately the same in countries with between 4 and 16 doctors per 10,000 people. It is a certain fact that while the number of patients treated by doctors is increasing in numerical terms, the number saved as a percentage of those who could be saved is falling dramatically. There are no signs of life expectancy improving in coming years.

2. The Protagonists

As a result of these disappointing figures many eminent observers both inside and outside the medical profession have begun to question medical priorities and, in particular, the value and relevance of work done by modern medical researchers. According to K. W. Newell, the Director of one division of the World Health Organisation, writing in the *WHO* Chronicle in January 1975, 'The rising costs of prevention, medical care and research and the decreasing quality and relevance of the services rendered are starting a whisper (which will probably later rise to a shout) to the effect that medicine is for the medical establishment and that there must be an easier and more effective way of solving the problems of heath.' The Director General of the World Health Organisation, Dr H. Mahler, presenting his 1974 Annual Report to the 28th World Health Assembly, made similar points: 'Conventional medical wisdom is being propagated as the only wisdom to growing numbers of people throughout the world, through both professional education and the mass information media. The issues at stake are not the scientific accuracy and technical proficiency of the methods used or those who use them, but the relevance of these scientific and technical endeavours to the solution of the critical health problems facing so many countries... Is it wise to devote so much effort to what are often only trivial advances in technical knowledge rather than to widening the range and measure the number of beneficiaries through the practical application of what is already known?'

Mahler went on to talk of the diminishing relevance of many of the more recent breakthroughs in medical knowledge. 'There are many roads to health,' he said, 'and most are paved with good intentions, but the most appropriate roads are not always those that have been charted by the medical cartographers.'

Lord Zuckerman has expressed a similar point of view: 'No one in his senses could suppose that with the world as it is, with most countries contending with a rate of population growth that threatens their economic and social development matters like the "in vitro cultivation of new human beings are a social necessity, or that the resources which they demand justify those extremes of surgical practice represented by techniques such as heart transplantation. These developments are the vested interests of medical or scientific enthusiasts not of the people at larger of social scientists or of governments.'

In his book *Reason Awake: Science for Man*, Rene Dubos quotes a British physicist, Professor Egan Crowan, as saying that 'The vast majority of the Earth's population regards science and technology as an increasingly mortal threat to their lives. They feel themselves powerless at the mercy of a few, as if they were on the operating table in the hands not of healers but of irresponsible playboys driven by curiosity.' As another scientist, quoted in the same book, put it, 'We may soon have to reconsider the wisdom of the traditional belief in the "duty" of science to explore the unknown unhampered by any other considerations.'

Similar sentiments were expressed by Selig Greenberg in *The Quality of Mercy*. He wrote, 'The greatest need today in the world's richest nation [America] is not for organ transplants or for some of the other marvels of the latest medical technology but for wider availability of the now commonplace results of the research of 25 or even 50 years ago.' Americans spend much more on acquiring new knowledge than on using what they have got.

The arguments put forward by those who oppose continued heavy expenditure on traditional types of medical research can be divided into several groups. A fundamental point rarely acknowledged by researchers themselves is that, as I shall show, future research programmes seem unlikely to be as productive as past research programmes. The cost of these doubtfully effective programmes is another problem frequently mentioned by the opponents of medical research. The same opponents often go on to argue that even if it were possible to discover useful information by routine research methods the possibilities are high that it will be far too expensive to implement the research findings. It is of relatively small economic importance to have to discard a chance discovery, but it may be an economic disaster to have to discard the results of a lengthy and expensive research programme.

There is undoubted evidence that much research is done for selfish reasons by narrow-minded researchers and there is additional evidence to show that the research they do merely causes confusion for practising clinicians and clogs up the communication channels which are intended to distribute useful medical information round the world.

Finally, there are a number of ethical arguments against the continuation of some research programmes. Opponents have attacked researchers both for the methods they have employed and for the ways in which they have presented their results. In particular, a number of doctors have complained that the application of recently developed techniques has damaged the infinitely valuable doctor-patient relationship and turned our hospitals into terrifying health factories.

Many scientists agree that research will not in future produce such important information as it has produced in the past. Dr Miles Weatherall of the Welcome Research Laboratories has pointed out that technical factors, legal limitations, emotional limitations, and financial limitations make progress on research in the pharmaceutical industry 'a whole lot more difficult'. Dr Weatherall put it simply: 'The easy discoveries have been made. It is the difficult ones that have been left.'

In a book called *Genes, Dreams and Realities*, published in 1971, Sir Macfarlane Burnet, who received the Nobel Prize for Medicine in 1960 and who had a long and distinguished career in medical research, said, 'The contribution of laboratory science to medicine has virtually come to an end ... Almost none of modern basic research in the medical sciences has any direct or indirect bearing on the prevention of disease or on the improvement of medical care.' Sir Macfarlane pointed out that scientific research 'employs a substantial proportion of the professional workers in any advanced country' and estimated that, in all, scientific research probably employs up to 5 per cent of a country's university graduates. He also made the point that, although the amount of competent scientific work being done is now enormous, the value of modern research work is often small: ' ... the new discovery, when it comes, usually has an air of triviality for any one not actually working in the field in which it has been made.'

Even some medical journals now seem to have doubts about the validity of the work they publish. According to an editorial in *World Medicine* in May 1975, 'For sheer volume of obscure triviality, the uncoordinated output of the cancer research laboratories takes some beating. For ponderous and jargon ridden dissertations on the self-evident, the literature of psychological research holds pre-eminence.' The writer of the editorial pointed out that 'Research is endowed with an aura of divinity. And we have become unconsciously the prisoner of the mentality that created it.' He argued that we should abandon many of our research projects and select with care those for further study. Sir George Pickering has written about the 'financial irresponsibility of those charged with supporting medical research' and has, as one of those responsible, confessed that he is now painfully aware of the fact that organising large-scale hunts for elusive answers is an unprofitable exercise. 'The master facts,' he has said, 'still escape us and they will be discovered, as they always have been, by chance and the prepared mind.'

Opponents of current medical research programmes also argue on financial grounds. Medical research, when it began in earnest, was often an amateur pursuit. It developed slowly in the nineteenth century as a part-time occupation, mainly of university teachers, and it became a full-time occupation for a few people only when research institutes were established privately and by governments in Europe and North America. Before the twentieth century medical research was usually the work of individuals, but in 1897 Frederick T. Gates, adviser to John D. Rockefeller on his philanthropic expenditure, said, 'Medicine can hardly become a science until it can be endowed and qualified men enabled to give themselves to uninterrupted study and investigation, on ample salary, entirely independent of practice.'

Today the total British expenditure on medical research is rather more than £100 million a year – a long way from the £55,000 spent on medical research in 1914. Even quite small trials can cost a great deal of money. The Royal College of Psychiatrists is said to have asked for £50,000 for a trial involving 200 patients, and Medical Research Council workers asked for over a million pounds to do a single trial on hypertension. Dr Paul Weiss, a biologist, and Dean of the Graduate School of Biomedical Sciences at the University of Texas, has complained about 'much shoddy, inconsequential, redundant, uncritical, and ill-conceived research, the mainsprings of which may have been nothing more than that "soft money" was available to support it'. In 1962 the American National Institute of Health returned 69.7 million dollars they could not get rid of and in

1963 they had a surplus income of 90 million dollars. In America one Congressional subcommittee has expressed concern over the fact that many of the people handing out research money in the States also do research and receive grants. It is not unknown for people to give themselves grants. Money does not get much 'softer' than that. The phrase 'medical research' has in fact become such a sure-fire money spinner in recent years that even the American Space Missions explained away their huge costs on the grounds that much of their work would be of medical value. They won public sympathy and support simply by claiming that sending men into space would help us cure the sick left behind.

It is not only research work itself which proves to be enormously expensive; the cost of applying what results may be obtained may well be prohibitive. As Enoch Powell has said in *A New Look at Medicine and Politics*, 'Every advance in medical science creates new needs that did not exist until the means of meeting them came into existence, or at least into the realm of the possible.' As we get richer and comparatively healthier, so our demands grow, our ability to accept discomfort falls and the expenditure on health rockets. There is no limit to the amount of medicine and medical care a population will absorb.

At a symposium organised by the drug company Roche, a Swiss speaker, Professor Alfred Pletscher asked, 'In a world in which hunger is rampant, in which treatable diseases remain untreated, in which the simplest of health care is lacking for millions, what are our justifications for those therapeutic measures that are so costly both in manpower and money?' He pointed out that a French economist had calculated that the cost of treating all patients needing artificial kidneys in France would equal the cost of all other health services in the country.

Rene Dubos put the same point in *Reason Awake: Science for Man*: 'One can anticipate the discovery of procedures for alleviating most human ills – drugs to correct physiological disorders or arrest infections; techniques for the removal, correction and transplantation of organs; development of mechanical prostheses for replacing diseased parts; and procedures for manipulating beliefs and moods. But it will probably be impossible in the foreseeable future to make the best methods of treatment available to all persons in need of them. No society, however prosperous and generous, will be able to carry the economic load and especially provide ·the large numbers of highly trained personnel that would be required to do all that could be and should be done.' If a cancer cure were found, we would probably not be able to afford to use it.

In a speech entitled 'Constraints upon the application of medical advances' given at the Royal Society of Medicine on 29 May 1974, Sir George Godber said that 'It is no longer possible to support everything which might lead to the increase of knowledge without regard to its applicability to the country's needs ... Not only is the potential demand for health care so great that it clearly could not be met even if all the funds demanded were available, but it is also beyond the potential development of trained staff.'

It has been suggested that much current medical research is done for the researchers' benefit rather than for the benefit of mankind. At a symposium organised by the Royal Society of Medicine, Professor Alan H. Williams of the Department of Economics at the University of York said, 'I suspect that far too much effort in medical advance is interpreted in the narrower sense and is directed at impressing the community of scholars. That is an important community, and one impresses it by research papers which lead to prestigious posts in well-endowed medical schools and a passport to the international congress jet set.'

The Director General of the World Health Organisation in an address to the 24th session of the WHO Regional Committee for Africa in September 1974 put the same point: 'Let us not forget that ... the major, and most expensive, part of medical technology as applied today appears to be more for the satisfaction of the health professions than for the benefit of the consumers of health care.'

Recognising that many scientists selfishly continue with work which interests them but which is unlikely ever to prove of value, Lord Rothschild, the author of the controversial Government report 'Framework for Government Research and Development', published in 1971, wrote that '... however distinguished, intelligent and practical scientists may be, they cannot be so well qualified to decide what the needs of the nation are, and their priorities, as those responsible for ensuring that those needs are met.'

Rothschild's idea was that, although scientists would have a chance to influence Government policy, politicians would have an equal chance to influence the work done by scientists and to direct scientists along channels likely to produce work of use to the community. However, after this report, there was a great outcry from scientists complaining that they were to be controlled by politicians.

One result of the report was that some of the money set aside for use by the Medical Research Council was directed to the Department of Health and Social Security. The hope was that the money would be spent more profitably. Unfortunately, the people who control the purse strings at the Department of Health seem to have no better idea of what research is likely to be of actual use than their counterparts at the Medical Research Council.

Researchers have also saturated our present communication media. According to Professor Jean Hamburger, Professor of Nephrology at the Faculty of Medicine of Paris, writing in the magazine *World Health* in September 1974, 'Even in a specialty as narrow as transplant immunology, for example, my laboratory has had to subscribe to 31 different journals from which in the last year alone we extracted, catalogued, and filed over 5,000 articles. In short, even the specialist is unable to keep pace with the growing mass of new data. Yet many of those data are vital if every patients to benefit from medical progress.' More than 40,000 reports were received by the WHO in 1974 from laboratories in the 43 countries cooperating with the Organisation in the collection and dissemination of information on viral infections. We cannot keep up with the results obtained by our researchers. Further new evidence is largely wasted and merely adds to the pile of unjudged, unused information in libraries and laboratories. '

Some opponents of medical research argue for the curtailment of current programmes on ethical grounds. They argue that medical research is likely to lead us into dangerous territory in the near future. Already it can be argued that we have changed our environment so drastically, multiplied our population so much, changed the nature of the human species so widely, that we already have little time left in which to find solutions to our self-created problems. Like the Irish elks who became extinct because of their hypertrophied antlers, homo sapiens may possibly become extinct because of his intelligence.

Medical research can also be described as being rather like a man running down a hill at greater and greater speed. He has to avoid obstacles and find a clear path as he accelerates downhill. So, it is with us. We have to research hard to find solutions to the problems our researchers have given us. Medical progress has changed the age structure of our society, giving rise to a whole new group of problems. Genetic research has already come a long way. According to Professor Salvador E.Luria, who gave a speech at a symposium organised by Roche, later published as *The Challenge of Life*, 'Once cloning becomes feasible the possibility arises that society, government or some other form of leadership will have the ability and the means of shaping people according to certain patterns; for work, for genius, for military purposes, for courage or for some other quality.'

Research into the brain is also progressing quickly. Dr Burgen, speaking at a Royal Society of Medicine Symposium said' ... we may be on the verge of understanding a whole new range of neuro-chemical functions that will permit much more specific handling of problems such as drive, concentration and learning ability.' Think of the ineffective and unsatisfactory way we have handled the problems created by transplants, artificial kidneys and so on and imagine how well we will deal with the ability to control human minds with some precision. Think of the disastrous way in which we try to deal with the problems we create for ourselves when we keep alive patients who will never regain consciousness.'

Practising clinicians are also saddened by the way in which the hospitals and clinics in which they work have been filled with pieces of machinery and emptied of caring people with time to spend on developing what used to be affectionately described as a 'bedside manner' but which today seems little more than a memory.

In his presidential address to the Association of American Physicians in 1975 (published in the October 1975 issue of *Archives of Internal Medicine*), David E. Rogers calls for technological restraint, pointing out that 'in our aggressive pursuit of precise diagnosis and with our vigorous therapeutic interventions we are sometimes going too far' and arguing that 'medicine, the physician, and the patient have lost something in the process.' He pleads for restraint and discrimination in the use of diagnostic and therapeutic methods, points out that in teaching hospitals patients often undergo arduous tests done to satisfy a specialist's curiosity, and clearly believes that the general internist, or general physician should conduct the orchestra of specialists and 'protect the patient from too much hazardous, wearing (and incidentally costly) investigation'. Despite this attack, Dr Rogers and his supporters make it clear that they applaud and appreciate the diagnostic and therapeutic technological advances of recent decades. Rogers is supported in an editorial entitled 'Evils of excessive application of technology in Medicine' which was published in the *Journal of the American Medical Association* in October 1975.

I have listed a good many of the arguments put forward by those who oppose spending money on medical research. There are, of course, a number of people who believe that we should continue to pump money and effort into medical research programmes, and who believe both that medical research has added considerably to the quality of life and that it will continue to do so in future years.

Some admit that the period of great discoveries is over but still argue that we should continue to hunt for new information. Dr A. S. V. Burgen of the National Institute for Medical Research was quoted at a Royal Society of Medicine symposium entitled 'Constraints on the advance of medicine' as saying, 'Without doubt the period of great growth is ended and the major concern is that the pace should not slow as a result of public indifference or aversion or the continuance of the mistaken view that more effort is needed in application at the expense of fundamental study.'

Some researchers support only the more practical programmes with obvious aims. Thus, for example, William H. Stewart, Surgeon General of the Public Health Service at the US Department of Health, Education and Welfare, in a paper entitled 'Research and public responsibility' argued, 'Research fields as rich in potential as the relationship between viruses and cancer, and developmental areas such as those related to the artificial heart and other organs merit and should receive special priority.'

Others believe firmly in the importance of basic research which has no immediate practical aims, but which is done in the hope that the knowledge obtained may prove useful at some future date. A. Landsborough Thomson, writing in *Half a Century of Medical Research*, said, '... research with an immediate object must necessarily draw upon the accumulated store of general knowledge and replenishes this only to a minor extent if pursued in isolation; the process is thus a self-exhausting one, and is rewarding only for a short period such as in wartime.' Writing in *The Lancet* in January

1971 Henry Miller said of basic research, 'It must be sustained on its own account and not, as sometimes happens, by spurious claims that it is likely to have early practical application.'

A few researchers seem to believe that their work is almost holy and therefore inviolable. Writing in the *New England Journal of Medicine* one researcher claimed that 'scientific research is the most powerful and productive of the things human beings have learned to do together in many centuries, more effective than farming or hunting and fishing or building cathedrals ... ' Others content themselves with trying to pour scorn and ridicule on those who would slow down research programmes. Professor Keith Reemtsma, an American transplant surgeon writing in the *Annals of Internal Medicine* put it this way: 'I do not doubt that the first caveman who trepanned a skull was assailed for trying an unproved operation, for proceeding without conclusive animal experiments, for forsaking the medical regimen of powdered owl feathers, for getting too much publicity, for siphoning off public funds for his work and denying support to the tiger-tooth necklace project, for interfering with the mysterious plans of the Great Spirit, and, of course, for prolonging the lives of unfit individuals and thereby placing in jeopardy the future of the Cro-Magnon race.'

Professor Reemtsma may mock the opponents of medical research programmes, but he has, like so many others who are involved in research, avoided answering any of these criticisms. The truth is, I fear, that many research programmes currently being financed are unnecessary, expensive and dangerous.

Habit, tradition, fashion, the inclinations of individual researchers and clinicians and the efforts of pressure groups all influence the directions in which medical research tends to drift. Research workers tackle problems they want to tackle, or problems they think they can solve. They do not choose problems which may need solutions outside the traditional schema of laboratory research. They ignore problems which may already have practical solutions. They search for answers we do not need to problems which do not matter, while answers we have to problems which do matter remain gathering dust in the libraries. Medical advances are not always advantages.

Many people have a vested interest in maintaining the status quo. There are hundreds of thousands of researchers earning a good living from the research industry and many thousands of clinicians making their way in the medical profession with the aid of research programmes they have initiated. Medical research is supported by the medical establishment in principle because research increases the demand for doctors and for medical aid in general. The more information we have and do not use, the greater the need for doctors and the greater the need for the services of the doctors we have. Factories do not want money taken out of pure medical research programmes because, if it is, it may well be pumped into preventive medical programmes which will undoubtedly mean big bills for industry. Companies that use unsafe manufacturing techniques, that produce dangerous products, that pollute the atmosphere, and so on, will all suffer if preventive techniques are perfected and made effective. If employers had to spend money on protecting workers, there would be less money to share out and wage rises would be smaller. The health care professions are also involved in what is effectively big business. In America the health industry employs over 36 million people with another million or so engaged in the production of drugs. In Britain the Health Service alone employs a total of nearly a million. Health care is one of the biggest and fastest growing industrial areas. Any change m emphasis would cause much disruption and arouse considerable protest.

To all this we must add the fact that professional and public expectations have been raised to great heights, that consequent public demands are enormous and that, as yet the profession and the public have not learnt to discriminate between useful and useless research work and medical care programmes.

Most doctors in clinical practice accept the myth that medical research still has much to offer. Their attitudes have been carefully nurtured over many decades by the researchers themselves (many of whom, resting comfortably on the achievements of their predecessors, think of themselves as rather superior beings), by academics who combine teaching with research and who find the quiet waters of research preferable to the hectic and often disturbed and disturbing waters of clinical medicine, and by doctors in practice who have been brought up to have nothing but respect and admiration for the medical researcher.

The public's attitude has been formed both by the medical profession and by science and medical writers anxious to provide their readers with hopeful and startling news. Initial scepticism which troubled the researchers of half a century ago has been replaced by an unreasonable and overwhelming faith that medical researchers will eventually produce all the answers and that spectacular cures are 'just around the corner'. Progress, the public is told, is part of human nature. So great is the public's faith in research that it is much easier for charitable organisations to collect money for research programmes than it is for them to collect money to provide medical and nursing care for the underprivileged sick.

Medical researchers have led us into a confused and confusing world where we no longer have either total free control over our own health or complete freedom to choose which avenues we wish to explore. The researchers have landed us with problems which we have to solve by accepting their solutions: in order to solve the problems created by doctors, we have to accept the solutions offered by doctors. And while we remain uncertain about what to do to solve these problems, the researchers fiddle happily in their laboratories. The scientists employed by our governments continue to look for simple answers to complex problems. The scientists employed by the pharmaceutical industry continue to produce marketable but medically unoriginal products which merely add to the world's problems rather than help to solve them.

We need to spend a few decades consolidating our position and tidying our base camp before we set off on any further exploratory missions. We need to assess our medical methods, we need to assess previously ignored and unfashionable techniques which may now have more to offer than traditional medicine, we need to study methods of dealing with the various personal and environmental pollutants which are such important causes of illness and death, and we need most of all to find solutions to the problems which our own researchers have created.

In the *Bulletin of the New York Academy of Medicine* in 1972 Dr N.R.E. Fendall wrote 'If I were asked to compose an epitaph on medicine throughout the twentieth century, it would read: brilliant in its discoveries, superb in its technological breakthrough, but woefully inept in its application to those most in need. Medicine will be judged not on its vast and rapid accumulation of knowledge per se but on its trusteeship of that knowledge.'

Speaking to a commemorative public meeting celebrating twenty years of the World Health Organisation, Lord Rosenheim said that we would make immense progress in health if within the next twenty years we could apply fully what we already know.

It is ironical that, when we have at last got the knowledge to help us ensure that medicine really does affect mortality rates for the first time in two centuries, we continue to search for answers which in reality we already have. Major causes of death in the younger age groups include cigarette smoking, various types of pollution, and accidents; and in the middle-aged groups, chest disorders, heart disorders and cancers. Most of these could be prevented if we applied the knowledge we have stored in our libraries.

It seems to me that one has to agree with the editorial writer in the *Medical Journal of Australia* who said in 1973, 'Medical research can no longer be allowed to grow at random, reacting only slowly and inadequately to the changing needs of community health and the ever-changing patterns of diseases.' For ethical, financial and common-sense reasons we must call a halt. As Theodor Fox put it in *The Lancet* in 1965, 'Today when so many progressive minds are preoccupied with ways of doing things, we too easily forget what ends these means are meant to serve.'

Meanwhile, however, the medical establishment is in the hands of the traditionalists-like the late Henry Miller, the medically qualified Vice Chancellor of the University of Newcastle upon Tyne, who, in his contribution to the book *Medical History and Medical Care*, published in 1971, wrote, 'Most of the diseases that are easily preventable are being prevented' and, in an attack on a physician who had expressed well-reasoned fears about the development of medical technology, said 'My impression is that he would prefer to be sick in a cottage hospital under the care of a physician in holy orders whose practice was uncomplicated by instrumentation of any kind.' Personally I am not at all convinced that I would prefer to occupy a bed in a modern, well-equipped hospital rather than an old-fashioned cottage hospital where tender, loving care is high on the list of priorities. It is, at the least, a choice which demands some consideration, and I hope that the rest of this book will provide the open-minded reader with much food for thought.

3. The Researchers

Within any research organisation, there will be a number of individual researchers who may be fired by personal ambitions as well as by the expressed intention of their employing organisation. This is true of all research organisations whether they be financed by government, by charity or by commercial companies.

To begin with, it is essential for a young doctor to do some original research if he is to become a success in his profession. The ambitious medical man must publish a paper or two or preferably more. Research work is therefore duplicated, with time, money and effort being wasted with no regard for the fact that all three are in short supply. The amount of money it costs young British doctors to do their research is incalculable. They are paid by the National Health Service, and they use National Health Service facilities, so on paper the research costs only the price of a stamp and an envelope to send the results off to a learned journal.

There are hundreds of small specialist journals in existence, each catering for a few hundred specialists, and making sure that each specialist can see his research work in print. It has been estimated that a new paper is produced every 26 seconds. That is not difficult to believe when one realises that in Britain alone there are approximately 150 journals for doctors, 36 of them called the *British Journal of* – There are such things as the *Journal of the British Society for Surgery of the Hand*! To keep a list of all these published papers is a full-time occupation for a number of people. Every month a book comes out called the *Index Medicus*. It is two inches thick, has 1.000 pages and contains nothing at all but the titles of medical research papers published throughout the world. In one recent issue, for example, there were no fewer than 75 papers dealing with potassium papers such as 'A study of the calcium, potassium and sodium content of toad atria'. From the *Index Medicus* it is easy to see that what is happening in Britain is happening all over the world. The research being done here is being duplicated in almost every other country. A conservative estimate is that 20 per cent of research work is unintentionally repeated by other workers.

The first scientific journals were published by the first scientific societies in the late seventeenth century and in those days, journals probably had far more readers than authors. Today, however, many journals have more contributors than sub scribers. (Many papers have several authors. I studied the *British Medical Journal* for 1973 and found that 1394 authors had written 426 papers.) One recent study showed that researchers seldom read the journals, but they are nevertheless anxious to publish in them. The journals do not survive on subscription fees paid by individual scientists but on a small number of inflated subscriptions paid by libraries which order and pay for the journals on the request of local scientists.

Within the medical profession, and indeed within all other branches of science, reputations are built, jobs obtained, and careers strengthened by the publication of scientific papers in the numerous journals. Dr R.R.M Porter, writing in the *British Medical Journal*, was blunt in his comments: 'In a committee advising on consultant appointments I have often been ridiculed when I have said that the main consideration should be the ability to treat patients skilfully. Research was invariably the deciding factor. I have known only two members of such committees who always took the trouble to read or look up the research articles written by the candidates.' In a paper published in the *Journal of Social Issues* in 1956 there was an analysis by Leo Meltzer of questionnaires completed by 75 per cent of all American physiologists. Meltzer found that 86 per cent of academic physiologists, 83 per cent of Government physiologists and 39 per cent of industrial physiologists said that they thought that published papers counted towards promotion. He also found that while more than half of academic and Government physiologists published more than five papers a year less than one-third of industrial physiologists published that many papers annually.

Speaking at a CIBA foundation symposium entitled 'Medical Research Systems in Europe' in 1973, George A. Smart of the British Postgraduate Medical Federation said, 'In some fields, though admittedly not in all, some research experience in a clinical research unit is considered essential for an appointment to a consultancy in the National Health Service. Once a consultancy has been obtained one incentive to engage in clinical research is a system of merit awards or "distinction" payments, and a considerable research output helps to gain the consultant such an award.'

George A. Smart also pointed out that doctors with private practice are also encouraged to do research work since, by having their work published m the Journals, they can gain the publicity which may bring them patients from all over the country.

There is an increase in the number of journals, the number of published papers and the number of lectures given each year. The volume of published research findings doubles every few years. The competition is so severe and the pressure on researchers to publish so continuous that many publish incomplete, badly presented and poorly judged work in journals which exist only because numerous libraries throughout the world pay the massive subscriptions charged. The pressures on researchers to get their work into print first is well illustrated in Paul Ferris's novel *The Cure*, about a team of cancer researchers, and in James D. Watson's book *The Double Helix*, the account of how Watson and his fellow-workers did the work on DNA which won them a Nobel Prize.

There is a strong incentive for researchers to conceal mistakes and adjust their experimental results and aims. Such occurrences are by no means uncommon, and the monk Mendel wasn't the only scientist to cook his results! The most recent scandal revolved round Dr William Summerlin who was brought to the Sloan Kettering Institute in New York at, according to Paul Ferris in *World Medicine* in August 1975, a salary of 40,000 dollars a year to do work on overcoming the rejection problems involved in transplanting skin. No other laboratories were able to duplicate Summerlin's work which had received a very high assessment from the American National Cancer Institute: but his achievement was only really questioned when he was found to have inked-in transplant sites with a black felt-tip pen on white mice supposed to have received transplants from black mice.

Summerlin's success, until his very obvious attempt to falsify his results was discovered, was not surprising when one reads the article entitled 'The Doctor Fox lecture: a paradigm of educational seduction' written by Donald H. Naftulin, John E. Ware Jr and Frank A. Donelly. An actor given the name of Dr Myron L. Fox was handed a few pages full of pseudo-scientific nonsense to recite to an audience of psychiatrists, psychologists, and teachers of medical subjects. All these people accepted the lecture happily, were pleased with it and when interviewed afterwards were convinced that they had learnt something and that they had read the publications of Dr Fox before!

In appreciation of the fact that the quality of scientific papers is more important than the sheer number of papers published, the *Scientific Citation Index* was founded in 1961. The compilers of the Index merely counted the number of times that each scientist was listed in the bibliographies at the end of the scientific articles. The theory was simple; the more important scientific work would be referred to more frequently than the work of minor importance. It was rightly estimated that scientists producing just one or two good papers would receive as high a citation rating as scientists producing whole batches of papers of less value. It was found that the list of most eminent scientists compiled in this way correlated well with a list compiled by scientists themselves and indeed with a list of Nobel Prizewinning scientists.

Unfortunately, the *Scientific Citation Index* is no longer considered quite so valuable. Scientists have discovered that a paper which describes a simple laboratory test which will be used in many other experiments will attract a great many citations. They have also discovered that a scientific paper which contains a mistake will be quoted frequently by other scientists anxious to correct the error. Cynics now say that the best way to get quoted regularly in the scientific literature is to write one or two papers full of outrageous mistakes.

A great many of the research papers written and published are valueless because the authors have been more concerned with the actual publication of papers than with the research work itself. In 1970 Herxheimer and Lionel, writing in the *British Medical Journal* reported on an examination of 141 reports of therapeutic trials published in four British medical journals. They found that one-third of these reports were quite unacceptable because they lacked one or more of the features required in a valid report. They were not convinced of the acceptability of another 16 per cent of the reports they studied. Some of the reports they looked at had poor or inappropriate methods of assessment, absent or inadequate controls and did not include all the necessary information.

The uncritical attitude of many researchers, desperate for publication credits to help them climb their career ladders, means that these points are often overlooked. It is understandably difficult for a young researcher to admit that many months, maybe even years, of work have resulted in nothing useful being proved. It is very easy for him to ignore the results which do not assist him in his attempts to reach a remarkable conclusion. Then, of course, the next researcher must follow a similar path if he is to reach similar conclusions.

It has been reported in the *New England Journal of Medicine* that the Chinese are considering publishing their medical journals anonymously, with articles published purely for their intrinsic worth. If we did this in the West the number of journals in existence would drop by at least 90 per cent and those remaining would shrink significantly in size. They would, however, still provide plenty of space for the speedy publication of those papers worth publishing.

It is not only for career reasons that scientists and doctors do medical research. Much of it is done for money and many doctors earn considerable sums of money by carrying out research programmes as well as their own clinical work. Despite rulings from most ethical bodies that researchers should not be paid for their work (since this effectively turns them into potentially biased employees of the people paying for the research), many are offered substantial sums to perform trials. A large number of doctors and scientists do indeed earn large sums of money this way.

The dangers of doctors being paid to do clinical research are well-illustrated by the case of Dr J.P. Sedgwick, a general practitioner working in London's West End. Dr Sedgwick was offered £10 per card to fill in a number of trial cards showing the effects of a new hypotensive drug on the blood pressure of some of his patients. Dr Sedgwick filled in 100 cards and accepted £1,000 from the company concerned, Bayer.

Bayer became concerned when the cards were returned, for not only were they still dean and unmarked, but the blood pressure figures (which all seemed to have been filled in at the same time) were identical on several sets of cards – a very unlikely occurrence! They reported the doctor to the General Medical Council and eventually, in July 1975, Dr Sedgwick had the dubious distinction of being the first medical practitioner to be struck off for such unprofessional behaviour. After the Sedgwick affair, when a Labour MP complained about doctors being paid to do trials, the British Medical Association defended the practice and a spokesman for the

Association of the British Pharmaceutical Industry said that the trials were organised by company trial experts.

It is not only individual researchers who are pressured and persuaded by money to do research which they, might not otherwise do. All research organisations are to some extent controlled by those who have to hand out the money. Industrial laboratories have, of course, to do research which is ordered by the board of directors and which relates to commercial requirements rather than clinical needs but Government laboratories are also influenced by financial factors. For example, because of public pressure, money is spent on cancer research. New research centres spring up because politicians want a centre in their own electoral area. In America black politicians have forced expenditure on sickle cell anaemia (a disease found only among blacks) to increase, and there have been similar rises in expenditure on Tay Sachs disease (which affects Jews) and Cooley's anaemia (which affects people of Mediterranean extraction). According to Henry Miller, writing in *The Lancet* in January 1971, ' ... positive direction of research is achieved by a variety of special organisations and pressure groups ranging from the tobacco industry to the Diabetic Association.' According to the Government publication *Health Trends*, Volume 7, 1975; 'For a disease affecting probably less than one person in 10,000, Huntington's chorea has prompted a surprising number of Parliamentary questions, and it has even been the subject of an Adjournment Debate.'

My comments will have probably surprised many who think of medical researchers as dedicated, brilliant people devoting their lives to science. I am afraid that it is not even true to describe all medical researchers as brilliant.

James D. Watson, one of the joint recipients of the Nobel Prize for Medicine and Physiology in 1962, wrote ' ... in contrast to the popular conception supported by newspapers and mothers of scientists a goodly number of scientists are not only narrow minded and dull, but also just stupid.' His claim is not only justified by the subjects researchers choose and the conclusions they draw but also by the ignorance they display when trying to study their results. The late Dr Richard Asher, a former consultant physician at the Central Middlesex Hospital, once wrote an article illustrating the illogical thinking of some researchers. He described how one researcher had reported that of 200 epileptic subjects 24 per cent had had infantile convulsions in the first two years of life while of 200 normal subjects only 2 per cent had had infantile convulsions. The man then concluded that a convulsion in the first two years of life suggests that the patient will develop epilepsy in later life and should therefore be treated with drugs, as if he were an epileptic. Undoubtedly this unknown researcher considered himself a saviour of the epileptic race. What he forgot, however, was that the incidence of epilepsy is 1 in 400 so, among 40,000 people, there would be 100 epileptics of whom 24 had infantile convulsions, while there would also be 800 normal people who had suffered from infantile convulsions. So those doctors who followed the dictates of this researcher would be treating 800 healthy people and 24 epileptics.

Another example used by Asher concerned the great Vitamin E mystery. Researchers have acclaimed those pregnant rats without Vitamin E miscarry and that therefore women who miscarry need extra Vitamin E, but there are more holes in this then there are in a string vest. We cannot, for a start, argue that because rats deprived of Vitamin E miscarry, giving rats Vitamins will prevent miscarriage, for that is like arguing that rats die without water and therefore giving them water makes them immortal. Then, who says that women are like rats when it comes to carrying babies. Are we to assume that everything that applies to the rat also applies to the human mother? Despite these holes in the argument researchers have recommended the use of Vitamin E and doctors have obediently prescribed it.

In this chapter I have painted a fairly bleak picture of the people doing medical research. I have concentrated on their shortcomings. Unfortunately, this chapter needed to be written because journalists and authors have in the past suggested that medical researchers are rather special people fired by special enthusiasms and not suffering from the usual human frailties. The truth is that as a group they are no different from any other group of professional workers. They have their own ambitions, fears and weaknesses, and these things influence the direction and quality of their research. They need also to influence our response.

4. Research in Progress

In 1870 the British Parliament approved a subsidy of 22,000 for scientific investigations. In 1914 a special Medical Research Committee was set up to handle funds of £55,000 a year allotted through the Government. Since those days the amount or money available has risen dramatically. The expenditure each year in Britain on medical research is now rather more than £100 million, having risen rapidly during the 1950s and 1960s. (In 1961/2 the Medical Research Council spent £5.5 million; in 1966/7 it spent £11.9 million.) This, however, is pocket money when compared to expenditure on medical research in the USA. There, money available to the National Institutes of Health for research totalled 701,800 dollars in 1945, 36,063,200 dollars in 1955 and 436,600,000 dollars in 1965.Since the end of World War II federal expenditure on medical research has multiplied 200 times and is still rising. Total expenditure on medical research in the USA rose from 160 million dollars in 1950 to 1,850 million dollars in 1965.

Money for medical research in Britain comes through four different types of agency. Firstly, there are the Government agencies such as the Medical Research Council and the Department of Health and Social Security which have a great deal of the taxpayers' money to spend on medical research. Secondly, there are the universities which are also financed by the taxpayers through the University Grants Committee and through other organisations. Thirdly, there are the industrial firms which pay for research in their own laboratories, in academic centres and in ostensibly private centres. Fourthly, there are the charitable organisations which receive money from subscriptions, donations, legacies and fundraising schemes. The charities have risen very quickly since the 1950s. Some give money to very specific projects designed to solve specific problems, others are more flexible.

According to an Office of Health Economics booklet, medical research is one of the fastest growth areas in terms of money spent in medicine. Money spent on medical research, for example, has increased at a faster rate than money spent on the National Health

Service. The trend seems to be towards a greater expenditure of money, through Government sources, though charities are also growing in size and in the amount of money they are distributing. In 1961/2 the amount of money spent on medical research by the Government was 58 per cent of the total, the drug industry spent 30.5 per cent and charities the other 11.5 per cent. By 1972/3 the Government share had risen to 61 per cent, the drug industry's share had fallen to 26.5 per cent and the charities' share had gone up marginally to 12.5 per cent. In 1961 the DHSS spent very little directly on medical research but by 1972 they were spending £10 million a year. After the publication of the Rothschild report suggesting that the DHSS should have more power over money spent on research, the DHSS has taken over part of the MRC's budget.

In recent years the Department of Health and Social Security has indeed become increasingly involved in research, being mainly and ostensibly concerned with practical, applied research and leaving basic research to the Medical Research Council. In the mid1960s the then Ministry of Health was spending three quarters of a million pounds on research, in 1971 it spent £5 million and in 1973 the level of expenditure had risen to £10 million although in addition the DHSS effectively had partial responsibility for the expenditure of a quarter of the Medical Research Council's allocation. This was forecast to rise to £19 million in 1974/5.

The Department's budget is intended to cover research into hundreds of problems concerning occupational health, environmental health, screening programmes, conditions of the elderly and so on, together with studies of how best to help the disabled and the mentally ill. Also included in the list of research projects for study are such problems of primary practice as deputising services, variations in hospital referral rates, variation in prescribing habits and variations in the use of diagnostic facilities. Then there are projects to study the development of invalid vehicles, artificial limbs, patient monitoring equipment and hearing aids.

The Medical Research Council was founded in 1913 and known at first as the Medical Research Committee. It had, and still has, a general responsibility for advancing medical Research in the United Kingdom, and it was expected to assess the total national effort and supplement this with such research projects as it thought necessary.

The Council has more recently given its aims as watching over the whole field of medical progress, supporting any promising research which needs support, coordinating the effort for the universities, the various government departments and the numerous other agencies involved in research work. Money is handed out in a number of ways. Researchers planning work which is intended to answer a single question or a small group of related questions may apply for a project grant which will provide funds for up to three years. Researchers interested in longer-term support can either obtain programme grants intended for research programmes with some broad objective, or they can work in one of the Council's official units.

During the 1950s and the 1960s, the years when the public (and its political representatives) still believed that anything spent on research would produce useful information, the Medical Research Council had little difficulty in providing funds for researchers. According to at least one commentator (writing in *World Medicine* in November 1974) there were often more funds available than there were people to use them.

In the financial year 1974/5 the Medical Research Council received a Parliamentary grant of £26 million; grants from other Government bodies (including the Department of Health and Social Security) of about £8 million together with other funds from private bodies brought the total income up to just over £36 million. The MRC on 1 January 1975 employed more than 4,000 people, of whom 304 were medically qualified, 748 were scientific staff, 1,665 were technical staff, 467 were maintenance staff and 883 were administrative and clerical staff.

The Medical Research Council not only gives grants to its own and outside research workers, but it also runs its own research centres. The National Institute for Medical Research is the largest of the Medical Research Council's establishments, having a rapidly rising budget which had at the last count reached about £3¼ million a year and a staff of 651. According to its own Annual Report, for 1973/4, `...the activities of the Institute cover a wide area of medical research and range from molecular and cell biology through to human physiology and field trials of chemotherapy in tuberculosis and leprosy, but since the Institute lacks clinical facilities, direct work on human problems is limited to that carried out in our Leprosy

Research Unit in Malaysia, and to collaborative work with clinical units elsewhere.' Perhaps the most interesting item from the Institute's annual report is the fact that the Animal Division which houses some 50,000 mice and 8,000 rats is producing 12,000 mice and 2,000 rats a month for research. Clinical work is done at the Clinical Research Centre, part of a general district hospital, Northwick Park Hospital at Harrow.

The Medical Research Council has been attacked for spending too much on basic research programmes and not enough on practical programmes. As a result its funds will in future be watched a little more closely, and a quarter of its budget will come via Government departments and will in theory have to be spent on genuine medical problems. Naturally, however, the Council still has its enthusiastic supporters. In an editorial written anonymously in the *British Medical Journal* in 1974 one writer complained, 'It has been said that the Council has committed too large a share of its resources to the disinterested unplanned research and not enough to the exploitation of new discoveries or to research on a consumer contractor basis. These criticisms are probably not widely supported.' The writer went on to comment on the MRC's achievements, flexibility, and lack of administrative clutter and to state categorically that 'the profession would deplore any serious changes in an organisation which has served it so well over the last 50 years.'

The function of the charitable organisations funding research programmes is said to be to fill the gaps left by the official organisations such as the Medical Research Council. This gives them a great deal of scope. They can certainly operate in areas where there are great public demands areas such as muscular dystrophy where many patients and their relatives are actively campaigning for more research. They can also begin programmes more quickly since there is usually less red tape to cut through before a research programme in a potentially interesting area can be got under way. Hopefully, there is also a greater chance that speculative ideas will be studied, though past experience does not totally support this view. The charitable groups sometimes provide money to those who have been rejected by official bodies because their work is highly specialised and likely to help only a very small minority, or because the work is a longshot gamble with a possibility of cure as the prize. In Britain

0.5 per cent of our Gross National Product is given to charity while Americans give 2 per cent.

In Britain alone there are scores of small organisations collecting money for medical research programmes and organising investigations into specific medical problems. These organisations vary in many ways. Some have very small fund raising organisations and manage their administration with the aid of voluntary helpers. On the other hand there are charitable organisations that collect and distribute millions of pounds each year and that operate with the aid of very professional advisers. In a later chapter in this book, dealing with cancer research, I discuss two large charitable organisations involved in the search for a cure for cancer.

Medical researchers, whether obtaining their funds from private or official sources, operate in many different areas of medicine. It would be literally impossible in a book of this length even to list the subjects being studied and the projects which are under way. There are several dozen recognised medical specialities and workers in every one of these branches of medicine are involved in research work.

It is difficult to decide which work in progress is likely to be of most value. Great advances certainly have been made in a few areas of research. For example, surgeons working in the field of restorative and cosmetic surgery have made considerable progress in the hundred years since Zielonko, a Russian pathologist working in Strasbourg, reported the first attempt to transplant autografts of skeletal muscle in the frog. In an article entitled 'A review of autogenous skeletal muscle grafts and their clinical applications' published in *Clinics in Plastic Surgery* in July 1974, a London surgeon, Noel Thompson, reported the use of extensor digitorum brevis muscles of the foot as grafts to reactivate paralysed eyelids.

Other work done by researchers, publicised as being of considerable value, has turned out to be of slighter clinical significance. For example, researchers recently announced that evidence suggested that multiple sclerosis might be caused by a virus. Despite the lack of firm evidence, the fact that the same suggestion had been made many times before, and the total lack of any possibility of the evidence leading directly to a cure, the discovery was given a tremendous amount of publicity by enthusiastic researchers and reporters, all of whom were guilty of the now common crime of raising the hopes of the sick and their relatives.

Some researchers are refreshingly honest about the real practical value of the work they do. Since 1946 scientists at the Common Cold Research Unit at Salisbury have been endeavouring to identify as many different kinds of cold causing virus as they can. The first efforts to find a cure for the common cold began in 1926 when Dr Alphonse Dochez and his colleagues in New York began the search. The Common Cold Research Unit, set up and paid for by the Medical Research Council and the Department of Health, has had visits by over 11,000 volunteers willing to help scientists find out more about the common cold. In his book entitled *In Pursuit of the Common Cold*, Sir Christopher Andrews, who helped set up the Unit, claims that its primary objective has been achieved: the improvement in our knowledge about the viruses which cause colds in man. He admits with remarkable honesty that it is unlikely that any cure will ever be found and suggests that the only real possibility is that some sort of prophylactic drug might be developed which could help people ward off colds.

Such honesty is rare, however, and many research programmes are planned and paid for without any thought being given to the possible value of any results or conclusions. Published accounts of Government sponsored research programmes, for example, show that many millions of pounds are spent on research which is highly unlikely to be of any clinical significance. Both the Department of Health and Social Security and the Medical Research Council, Britain's major promoters of Government sponsored research, publish fairly detailed reports which show that it is Government research which is least likely to prove useful.

For example, a great deal of the money allocated for medical research by the Department of Health and Social Security is spent on projects of doubtful value. The Atomic Energy Research Establishment at Harwell, for instance, has received a grant of £135,000 for the development of nuclear-powered batteries for cardiac pacemakers. Unfortunately, the National Health Service is so short of money that such batteries are unlikely to be available for many years. A great deal of money has been spent on research into computerised transverse axial tomography of the head 'to identify positions and natural space occupying lesions' but the machinery needed to use these techniques is too expensive for the Health Service.

Over a million pounds were allocated in the year 1971/2 to the South Western Regional Hospital Board who were apparently attempting to develop a computer system which would enable all medical, nursing and administrative staff to have convenient access to patients' records. In the same financial period the Microbiological Research Establishment at Porton Down received a grant of £835,000 from the Department of Health and Social Security.

A great deal of money is spent each year on sociology projects: there was a grant of £21,000 to social workers at the University of Leicester for a study entitled 'Coloured children in care', and a grant of £17,000 was given to Reading University for a series of projects, including one entitled `Why staff leave the Reading hospitals'. There was a grant of £61,00 to the Tavistock Institute of Human Relations' Centre for Applied Social Research, for a project entitled `The development of self-innovation in hospitals through the aided use of social research'.

There were a number of very introspective sociology studies being funded. Dr K.A. Hack of the Department of Economics and Social Science at the City of Birmingham Polytechnic is listed as having had £600 for a project designed to facilitate the task of those who interview applicants for social work courses, and the Department of Sociology and Social Administration at Southampton University received £22,400 for a ' Study of social service departments' .

A sum of £3,000 was allocated to University College, London, where the aim of the project was said to be 'to establish a method of understanding the process by which the need for bodily nutrition is harnessed to the demands of the social system. Taking the family unit as a gastronomic community, an attempt will be made to identify the boundaries of intimacy and distance expressed by food sharing and food exchanging in four families.' And there was £11,000 for the `Evaluation of the general management development courses for senior Health Service managers' at the School of Management Studies at the Polytechnic of Central London.

One wonders at the wisdom of the administrators with the purse strings who give f1 1,800 for the 'Study of the prevalence incidence morbidity and mortality of heart block and bradycardia in the Devon clinical areas'; £28,000 for a study of 'Attempted suicide in the Oxford region'; £243,000 for research aimed at helping to train dentists in the use of dental auxiliaries and a mere £2,500 spread over the years 1971/4 for 'Projects concerned with the safety of medicines'.

According to the description of research programmes financed through the Department of Health and Social Security, research by nurses is becoming increasingly popular. The General Nursing Council has a research unit which in 1971/2 received £20,000 for projects such as 'Career pattern study of newly qualified nurses' and 'Analysis of applications and admissions to experimental schemes of nursing education'. The Department of Social Administration at the University of Hull received £16,000 for a 'Survey of male entrants to nursing' Since they found a total of 542 male nurses to study, this means that the survey cost about £30 a nurse. A grant of £10,900 was awarded to R.A. Pinker at the Department of Sociology at Goldsmiths' College for a study entitled 'Towards an understanding of nursing' and there was a grant of £16,200 to the University of Wales for a study on 'Role conflict among student nurses'.

In 1973/4, according to the official publication 'Health Trends', the amount spent by the Department of Health and Social Security on centrally financed research into medical equipment and hospital supplies was a total of £1,694,000. Of this sum a mere 16 per cent was spent on work associated with equipment and aids for the disabled. In the same financial year the DHSS spent £304,000 on research and development of health services planning and organisation, and £292,000 on research into staffing problems within the Health Service and the Social Services (the title of the research was 'Quality and quantity of resources manpower and training').

The expenditure on studies involving environmental health, on the other hand, came to a miserly £41,000 – a sum which hardly supports the official suggestion that even if the Medical Research Council does not make sure that the research it finances is what the people need, at least the DHSS tries to ensure that some practical research is done.

As a writer in the *British Medical Journal* put it in June 1974 '...it is far from clear at present what the Department's policy is; for example, it has been financing 56 projects concerned with technology and hardware and 40 using computers as against only 8 dealing with handicapped children.'

The latest edition of the Medical Research Council's annual report supports the theory that the MRC is also still spending most of its money on basic research rather than on useful practical research. They set up in April 1974 an MRC Mammalian Development Unit at a cost of £52,376 with the aim of obtaining an understanding of the factors regulating growth and development in the mammalian embryo. The Brain Metabolism Unit received in 1974/5 a sum of £226,692, the Cyclotron Unit £877,554, the National Institute for Biological Standards and Control £986,373, the Unit on the Experimental Pathology of the Skin £110,129, the Lipid Metabolism Unit £103,088, the Medical Sociology Unit £110,181, the Mineral Metabolism Unit £196,767, the Radiobiology Unit £631,420 and the Reproduction and Growth Unit £144,140. The MRC Molecular Genetics Unit received £90,167, the Laboratory of Molecular Biology received £1,561,384 and dozens of other projects in the field of genetics received large grants. The MRC Laboratory Animals Centre received a massive £318,268.

In contrast to this wild expenditure on basic research projects which have little or no bearing on the problems of our patients, the Medical Research Council's Unit for Physical Aids for the Disabled received a grant of £5,934. According to the MRC's 1974/5 Annual Report, 'Accidents are the commonest cause of death between the ages of 1 and 40 and are the third commonest cause, after ischaemic heart disease and cancer, of death during working life. They are also an important cause of both minor and severe disablement.' I suppose we should be grateful that the MRC at least acknowledges where our real problems lie. They do little about it, however, and their spending on research in this area is as derisory as their expenditure on physical aids for the disabled.

In view of the MRC's apparent lack of interest in any subject of positive clinical value, I was pleasantly surprised to read in the summer of 1975 that Dr Lever, the Director of the Medical Research Council's Blood Pressure Unit, had indicated that the MRC was asking the Department of Health for between £1 and £2 million (research workers are traditionally vague when asking for money) to fund a survey into the treatment of high blood pressure. Considered to be probably the most expensive medical survey ever to be conducted in Britain, the study would try to find out whether or not there was any medical value in treating patients with mild blood pressure problems. The study would involve between 20,000 and 40,000 patients (the vagueness here may or may not be related to the vagueness in relation to the estimated cost of the exercise), half of whom would receive a hypotensive drug for five years and half of whom would receive a placebo for five years.

Since general practitioners write about six million prescriptions a year for hypotensive drugs and since those drugs cost the National Health Service rather more than £10 million a year, it would certainly be useful to know if the treatments presently being offered are useless. Equally it would prove embarrassingly expensive if the trial showed that all people with moderately raised blood pressure should be treated, since one estimate is that 15 per cent of all middle-aged Britons might well have hypertension.

There are unfortunately a number of questions which must first be asked about such a trial. The obvious question is how one can justify giving placebos to patients for five years. Inevitably tablet taking is a nuisance and a worry. The patients involved must be convinced that they need medication (if the placebo is to do its job) and will have to spend a good deal of time visiting their general practitioner for the sake of medical science rather than any benefit to themselves.

The other obvious question is, why should it cost so much money simply to give drugs and placebos to patients and keep a record of their blood pressure and general health? If we assume that a trial involving 20,000 patients is going to cost £1 million, it is not difficult to determine that, since the trial is expected to last five years, the organisers are planning on spending £10 a year on studying each participant. Since the general practitioner receives only about £2 a year to provide total medical care for each person on his list, it is difficult to understand why an MRC Unit should receive £10 for doing rather less work. Indeed, I cannot understand why such a project, if it is necessary and worthwhile, should cost more than the expense of printing a few extra forms, collecting them and feeding the results into a computer.

In1950 the MRC spent £200,000 on building a cyclotron at Hammersmith Hospital. They treated about 100 patients there in two decades and then ordered a second cyclotron, to be built in Canada, intended for use in Edinburgh in 1976. The cyclotron projects a neutron beam which is said by its supporters to damage cells and to therefore be a useful tool with which to kill tumours. It is a marvellous sounding piece of equipment but an article written on behalf of the MRC and appearing in *Health Trends* 1974, admitted that '... unfortunately it has not so far affected survival figures since the patients have mostly died from metastases [secondary tumour sites].' The cost of the Edinburgh cyclotron was estimated to be about £800,000 and was compared in one medical journal with the expenditure of money on Concorde: 'Concorde and the cyclotron alike represent largely irrelevant responses to our needs.'

Some of the MRC's other expenditures have also had their critics. The Council's headquarters are in a most expensive part of London the W1 postal district. There is no real reason why the headquarters should not be in the Midlands or the North of England, where property is cheaper.

The money wasting might perhaps be forgivable if there had been some spectacular results. But there have not. The MRC did manage to develop a miniature tape recorder small enough to be worn by the patient and to record the ECG continuously for up to three days, and it has also produced an allegedly original solution to the problem of how to treat the overweight: a solution involving the use of a dental splint to keep the jaws fixed together.

I have listed and described a number of research projects which are, in my view, of little real value to practising detours on their patients. There are, in addition, many research projects being financed which are unlikely to be of any value at all!

In the *British Medical Journal* in November 1975, for example, there was a paper entitled 'Changes in breast volume during normal menstrual cycle and after oral contraceptives', written by a scientist from the Department of Zoology at the University of Edinburgh and two scientists from the Medical Research Council's Unit of Reproductive Biology in Edinburgh.

Four girl volunteers, all aged 21, were used. Their left and right breasts were measured daily by the Archimedean technique of placing a glass mixing bowl seven inches in diameter inside a larger container and then filling it with water. The girls then knelt on the floor over the mixing bowl and lowered first the breast and then the other into the bowl, thereby displacing pater which overflowed into the container. The water which was displaced was measured afterwards.

Measurements were taken daily for three months, using water of the same temperature, and three consecutive measurements were taken to ensure accuracy. Studies were done to find out whether or not a girl's previous posture affected her breast volume. For example, breast sizes were assessed after the owners had been lying down for four hours and for 11½ hours, and then after the owners had been standing up for four hours and for 11½ hours. The researchers found that the girls breasts seemed to shrink when they were immersed in cold water and that girls who had been standing up for long periods had bigger breasts than they had when they had been lying down.

Since only four girls were used in the experiment, since it must be difficult, if not impossible, to decide where a chest wall stops and a breast begins, and since there is a considerable amount of breast tissue in the chest wall, the purpose of this experiment escapes me completely. It sounds fun to do but can have no real scientific value.

The same is true of a study on the anthropometry of airline stewardesses in the United States which was carried out for the Federal Aviation Administration, who paid out £26,000 to the researchers. The study involved the researchers in taking 79 different measurements on a total of 423 girls. As well as the more usual measurements such as height, weight and bust size, the researchers took measurements to find the knee to knee breadth while sitting, the height of the nose, the maximum horizontal width of the jaw and the length of the buttocks.

The object of the exercise was said to be to help with the design of aircraft furniture but one wonders how helpful it was to find out that the average airline stewardess is between six stone eight pounds and ten stone five pounds, between five feet tall and six feet tall and measures between 29-21-29 and 38-28-38 in the places where women are usually measured.

There is, of course, research work which does add to our stock of useful information. Researchers developing new surgical techniques, new drugs and new pieces of diagnostic equipment are undoubtedly producing some useful information. What I question is the value of the results when one considers the costs; in addition, I also suspect that the problems produced by much current medical research are considerable.

To illustrate research work being done, to describe why I think much of it is likely to produce more problems than it solves, and to help explain why we should be suspicious and even frightened of the activities of our medical researchers, I have chosen to write very briefly about four different aspects of medical research.

The branch of medical research which attracts most money, publicity and glamour is cancer research and so I begin with a description of cancer research programmes in existence. Genetic research is one of the fastest growing branches of medical research and one which is said by some to offer the most and by others to be the most frightening. This will be the second general aspect of medical research described. Since Christiaan Barnard performed the first heart transplantation, the replacement of diseased organs with new ones has attracted a great deal of public acclaim and criticism. It may seem strange to describe transplantation as 'research' rather than treatment' but few thinking clinicians regard it in any other way. This will be the third aspect of research discussed. The fourth subject I have chosen to write about is also one very much in the public eye and one very much likely to become increasingly important in future years: research into mental problems.

These are the topics discussed in the following four chapters.

5. Cancer Research

Since approximately 180,000 new cases of cancer occur each year in the United Kingdom and about 130,000 people die each year from one or other of the various types of cancer, and since cancer is responsible for about 20 per cent of all the deaths in the United Kingdom, it is hardly surprising that there are two big charitable organisations taking money from British people for work intended to reduce those figures. The Imperial Cancer Research Fund and the Cancer Research Campaign both have incomes running into several million pounds.

Of these two charitable organisations the Imperial Cancer Research Fund is the older. It supports cancer research principally in its own establishments, its main laboratories being in the expensive Lincoln's Inn Fields.

In the second decade of the twentieth century some surgeons, pathologists and clinicians began to feel that cancer research as done in the Imperial Cancer Research Fund's own laboratories was not attacking the problem adequately. In 1923 Sir Richard Garton, an industrialist, provided £20,000 to set up the British Empire Cancer Campaign (now called the Cancer Research Campaign). Like the ICRF, the CRC spends a good deal of the money it raises from the public on its own laboratories but it does also spend money on supporting researchers in hospitals and universities.

There has always been some rivalry between these two huge organisations and, despite the fact that since 1970 there has been a Cancer Coordination Committee with members from the MC, the CRC and the ICRF, much money must have been wasted in the last half century on unnecessarily duplicated work.

In 1974 the Cancer Research Campaign had an income of over £4½ million. In 1937 the income had been £37,000, in 1957 it had reached £¾ million, in 1972 it was £3 million and in 1973 it was £4 million. Critics do not find it difficult to argue that the Campaign is hardly spending its money wisely. According to the introductory statement to the 52nd Annual Report for 1974, written by His Grace the Duke of Devonshire, the Chairman of the Campaign, the CRC has recently undertaken the purchase of a good deal of expensive equipment to help 'to maintain Britain's place in the forefront of radiobiological research'. This included a sum of £350,000 spent on a cyclotron for the University of Edinburgh. The Campaign has also spent money on supporting academic workers. It has, for example, established a Chair of Clinical Oncology and Radiotherapeutics at the University of Cambridge for Professor N.M. Bleehen, formerly Head of the Department of Radiotherapeutics at the Middlesex Hospital Medical School. The CRC gave £275,000 to establish this chair and according to His Grace's comments, this will `provide for the salary of the Professor and his secretary'. The Medical Research Council are apparently paying the costs of the rest of the staff and the running costs for the Unit.

In addition, in 1974 the Cancer Research Campaign paid for 41 delegates to attend the 11th International Cancer Congress in Florence, spending a total of £10,695 or about £250 per delegate. As one contributor to the CRC's Annual Report was honest enough to put it, `No doubt the site of the Congress contributed to the size of the attendance. Those who have held collecting boxes on rainy days will be pleased to note that the Mayor's cocktail party for the delegates was held in some ancient cloisters and that the delegates seem to have had a splendidly luxurious time. Altogether, the Campaign spent over £25,000 on sending delegates to meetings.'

Like the Cancer Research Campaign the Imperial Cancer Research Fund seems to spend most of its money on long-term projects. The ICRF employs a huge staff of scientists though few have any medical qualifications. According to the ICRF's 1974 Scientific Report, 'Much of the research at Lincoln's Inn Fields and Mill Hill continues with the long-term aim of explaining in molecular terms the change from a healthy cell into a cancer cell, with its abnormal growth and invasive properties.' Much of the ICRF's scientific work is so esoteric that it is difficult for the onlooker to relate it to the problems of those patients with cancer. The Scientific Report contains details of such studies as 'Complex carbohydrate containing macromolecules at the surface of hamster cells in culture' and `Effects of age and carcinogen treatment on epithelial mitotic activity in organ culture of adult mouse colon' There is no real evidence to show that the results of work on animals are of use when treating human beings. The Imperial Cancer Research Fund has an income of £5¾ million.

When the ICRF was founded in 1902 by the Royal College of Physicians and the Royal College of Surgeons, the first director made a plan of attack for the Fund. The writer of the 1974 Annual Report proudly tells readers that this plan is still being followed. One might think that since it has proved singularly unsuccessful, the time might have come for a change of attitude.

Medical researchers involved in publicly or charitably financed cancer research persist in looking for the 'magical cure'. There are a number of favoured areas. Some workers believe in immunotherapy, others in radiotherapy and yet others in chemotherapy. One drug recently given the headline treatment turned out to have been tested on a grand total of 19 patients. The statistical value of such a small study is minute.

One of the most expensive and prestigious projects is the use of neutrons in the treatment of some cancers. Since 1971 workers at the Hammersmith Hospital in London have been busily studying the effects of fast neutrons on tumours of the head and neck. The first results of the project were published in the British Medical Journal in June 1975 and entitled, First results of a randomised clinical trial of fast neutrons compared with X or Gamma rays in treatment of advanced tumours of the head and neck.' The article was written as a report to the Medical Research Council which had funded the project. The researchers were presumably hoping to show the superiority of neutrons but unfortunately by June 1974, 25 of the 52 neutron-treated patients had died and 30 of the 50 X or Gamma ray-treated patients had died. For some reason or other, later mortality figures were not available in the summer of 1975.

Much laboratory work has been started on the mistaken assumption that there is one disease called 'cancer' and that there will be a cure' which will enable doctors to treat all patients suffering with cancer. Many projects have been funded because organisers (both qualified and lay) have believed that they might solve the problem of cancer once and for all to the well-publicised credit of everyone concerned. Much money has undoubtedly been wasted on research which has duplicated work done elsewhere and which has moved in directions unlikely ever to prove of practical benefit.

One of the most important breakthroughs in cancer research of recent years was made, not by researchers in expensive institutes, but by a practising British surgeon, Denis Burkitt. working in Uganda. His first research grant from Government funds totalled €15 and his second, for £150, came from the Medical Research Council and was spent on an old jeep. By logical, patient study Burkitt managed to map the occurrence of a tumour common in children in that part of the world. He matched the map he prepared with other factors and eventually managed to show that the cancer was probably caused by a virus. Eventually he learnt how to cure the tumour. So, one of the most important discoveries was made, not by a professional researcher but by an observant doctor happy to continue his studies in his own time and at his own expense. Too many doctors these days are unwilling to begin any research programme unless they are first financed by an official agency and properly recognised as bona fide research workers.

The total expenditure on cancer research may seem large in Britain but it is minute when compared with the expenditure in the United States. In January 1971 President Nixon called for a total national commitment to find a cure for cancer. The Cancer Act of 1971 provided for an increase in the financial allocation to the National Cancer Institute which is part of the National Institutes of Health but which has an independent director. Nixon made 440 million dollars available for cancer research in 1972/3 and planned to make 1,000 million dollars a year available by 1980. America spends three or four times as much on biomedical research per head of population as Britain does.

The first steps for the creation of a practical National Cancer plan were taken in 1970 when 250 specialist scientists came together, partly under the auspices of the National Cancer Institute, to help rationalise cancer research. They aimed to list scientific and medical problems to be solved and to choose objectives for future research, although, as some critics pointed out, it is often difficult to tell which research is relevant and usually impossible to pick out research projects likely to prove fruitful in the future.

Similarly enthusiastic programmes are going on in other parts of the world. In 1963 thirteen distinguished French intellectuals, including the ubiquitous Jean-Paul Sartre, appealed to General de Gaulle, asking that one half per cent of the military budgets of the

USA, USSR, UK and France be made available for the financing of various aspects of medical research. In 1964 President de Gaulle asked the USA, USSR, UK, Italy and Germany to join France and contribute one half per cent of their Defence Expenditure each year to an international effort to conquer cancer. They formed together the International Agency for Research in Cancer, with headquarters in Lyon under the control of the World Health Organisation; and this Agency, which today receives over £100,000 from the UK each year, is now busy organising international epidemiological studies. It was officially established by the 18th World Health Assembly and receives financial support from Australia, Belgium, the Federal Republic of Germany, Japan and the Netherlands as well as the other countries I have mentioned.

Throughout the world many hundreds of millions of pounds are spent every year on cancer research. The annual total expenditure is probably close to £1,000 million. And by no means all doctors or lay observers are convinced that this massive expenditure is justified.

An American science writer, Daniel S. Greenberg, contributing to the *Columbia Journalist Review* early in 1975, used figures which he obtained from the National Cancer Institute in the USA to question the efficiency of cancer research. He pointed out that, according to these statistics (the figures with which cancer workers originally hoped to be able to persuade the rest of us that they were winning the battle), from 1940 to 1949 the five-year survival rate for patients with lung cancer (something like 10 per cent of all cancers) was 4 per cent; that the five-year survival rate rose to 8 per cent between 1950 and 1959 and then rose again, but to only 9 per cent between 1965 and 1969. The five-year survival rate for patients with cancer of the colon has not improved at all since the 1950s and the one-year survival rate for cancer of the colon seems to be actually falling. Cancer of the cervix carried a 59 per cent survival rate in the years 1950/59 and the survival rate per cent was only 56 in the years 1965/9.

The five-year survival rate for acute leukaemia, on the other hand, has risen from 1 per cent to 3 per cent and there have been a number of individual success stories. Even here, however, the general story is not one of a victory. The advances which have been made, usually involving the use of powerful drugs in combination, have often proved specific for particular varieties of leukaemia. Spectacular advances have been made in the treatment of one or two rare childhood leukaemias, for example; but, sadly, these advances have only helped a few dozen children. There are many different varieties of leukaemia and doctors involved in this area of research have to continue experimenting with new drug combinations, treating perhaps half a dozen patients with one combination and another half a dozen patients with a fresh combination. No major breakthrough seems possible with the present techniques.

In addition there is the problem that the compounds on which the cancer-killing drugs are based are toxic not only to cancer cells but also to normal tissues. So the drugs cause many painful and uncomfortable side-effects.

Some scientists argue that the early improvement in the figures for the 1950s was due more to the introduction of antibiotics and blood for transfusions than to better methods of treating the cancer. In other words, patients recovered from surgery because of improved surgery techniques. These improvements would have come without cancer research programmes. Certainly the latest American figures, which show that in the first seven months of 1975 there was a 5.2 per cent increase in the number of deaths from cancer compared to a 1 per cent increase in other recent years, are discouraging.

Nor do British statistics suggest that much progress has been made in the battle against cancer. In the age group 65 to 74 the death rates per 100,000 male members of the population were 1,053 in 1950 and 1,336 in 1972. Cancer of the lung and cancer of the breast are more common now in men and women in the age groups 45 to 64 than they were in 1950. Death rates per 100,000 people have risen significantly. The five-year survival rate for cancer of the stomach was about 11 per cent in 1948 for both men and women. Figures in the late 1960s showed that the five-year survival rate had fallen to about 6 per cent. According to the *Cancer Handbook of Epidemiology and Prognosis* published in 1974 by Churchill Livingstone and compiled by J.AH. Waterhouse, Director of the Birmingham Regional Cancer Registry and Reader in Medical Statistics at Birmingham University, the five-year survival rate for patients with cancer of the stomach has now fallen to between 4 and 5 per cent. Five-year survival rates for patients with lung cancer, cancer of the cervix and cancer of the uterus have hardly altered in the same period.

The five-year survival rate for British women with breast cancer has fallen from 53 per cent to 49 per cent in the same period. In the *British Medical Journal* of May 1972 an editorial writer complained that 'there is more controversy about the management of breast cancer than almost any other topic in tumour therapy'. The writer went on to point out that many different types of operation, ranging from simple removal of the lump to the removal of the whole breast and all surrounding lymph glands were being done and that '.. each of these diverse treatments has its fervent advocates, and yet despite a plethora of reports there is little evidence on which to recommend as the best buy for the patient.' Not even controlled trials seem to have helped for, according to the BMJ, writer, 'the choice of treatment has had little effect on survival'.

The cancer researchers can hardly claim any great benefits from their work in this field. Even the usually conservative World Health Organisation came out in July 1975 with a statement headed 'Breast Cancer – 50-year statistics show no improvement' and said that 'Present methods of treatment do not seem to be having any overall impact upon the disease or upon the heavy toll it takes of female lives.'

In no country in the world is there any evidence of a decline in mortality from cancer of the breast, even when figures are adjusted to allow for the fact that the female population includes more older members today. Statistics show an increase in mortality in the last 20 years in both the USA and England.

Even more telling, however, is the argument put forward by the epidemiologists who have shown that there has been for many years a strong correlation between the development of cancer and the exposure to chemical substances of one sort or another.

In 1775 a prominent English surgeon, Percival Pott, described cancer of the scrotum in chimney sweeps. Since then many other occupational and environmental relationships have been found. It has been proved that wood can cause cancer of the nasopharynx and cancer of the sinuses, that tobacco causes cancer of the tongue, pharynx, lung and oesophagus, and that alcohol causes cancer of the oesophagus. Diets low in fresh vegetables and fruit are likely to result in cancer of the stomach. Occupational cancers are common these days because of new methods of manufacture, waste disposal, power production and food processing. Rubber workers are in danger of developing bladder cancer and workers exposed to cutting oil are particularly likely to develop skin cancers. Sadly, this list expands month by month.

The introduction of synthetic chemicals into such things as pesticides, agricultural preparations, food additives and cosmetics means that many millions of people may be exposed to harmful carcinogenic substances.

In an article entitled `Do hair dyes cause cancer?' published in *World Medicine* in autumn 1975, Colin Tudge points out that according to Bruce N. Ames and his colleagues at the University of California, about 90 per cent of oxidative-type commercial hair dyes are mutagenic. That is to say, they have a fair chance of being carcinogenic or causing cancers to develop. Three-quarters of the 250 million-dollar-a-year American hair dye market is concerned with the oxidative type of hair dyes. According to Ames, about 30 per cent of American women dye their hair every month. (One has to remember that a compound with a 1 in 10,000 chance of causing cancer could cause several thousand cancers in Britain alone, if such a large proportion of the population were exposed.)

The problems created by chemically induced cancers were discussed in `Health Trends' in August 1975 by Dr Carter and Dr Symington, respectively Professor of Pathology and Director at the Chester Beatty Research Institute, London, who agreed that over 70 per cent of human cancers are probably wholly or partly caused by chemicals. They showed that despite the well-known historical association between soot and scrotal cancer, there are still cases of cancer caused by similar substances. For example, the Birmingham Regional Cancer Registry recorded 187 cases of scrotal cancer between 1950 and 1967 and at least two-thirds of these men had worked with mineral oils. Mineral oil mists have also been listed as causes of scrotal cancers among lathe workers. The Manchester Regional Cancer Registry, for example, has reported a high incidence of scrotal cancer among lathe workers.

Carter and Symington also report that there is now evidence that exposure to tar fumes is also linked with the development of cancer. Studies among British gas workers have, they claim, shown an increase in the incidence of lung cancer, cancer of the bladder, cancer of the skin and cancer of the scrotum. An increase in the incidence of lung cancer has also been reported from doctors studying gas workers in North America.

Workers in paint factories, textile factories, printing works, and in work involving the use of tar, pitch and gas are at risk from other substances which have in recent years been shown to act as carcinogens, Workers in chemical, rubber and cable making industries are also listed as being at risk. Carter and Symington assert that in some industrial communities the incidence of occupational bladder cancers may be running at about 20 per cent.

The manufacturing processes used in the preparation of polyvinyl chloride (PVC) have been unchanged for several decades, but it was not until 1974 that it was shown that workers in the industry were developing liver cancer. Work done in the United States, Great Britain, Scandinavia, West Germany, France, Italy, Romania and Czechoslovakia has supported this observation. Workers involved in using asbestos have a greater chance of developing lung cancers, as do workers exposed to small amounts of arsenic.

The evidence is so convincing that most experts believe today that the great majority of cancers are caused by chemical substances of one sort or another. According to the International Agency for Research on Cancer (an independently financed organisation which is effectively a part of the World Health Organisation) 80 per cent of all cancers are environmentally induced. The Director of the American National Cancer Institute has publicly stated that he believes that the figure is nearer to 90 per cent. Eric Boyland, for many years Professor of Biochemistry at the Institute of Cancer Research in London, concluded after careful consideration of all the likely causes of cancer that between 85 and 90 per cent of all human tumours are caused by chemicals. According to the 1974/5 Annual Report of the Medical Research Council, 'This statement has never been seriously challenged and the experience and research of the past few years has tended to support this view of cancer.' Dr David Baltimore a Nobel Prize-winner for Medicine is reported to have claimed that the increase in the incidence of cancer in our society reflects the environmental changes of the last half century.

If we took the advice given by the experts who quote these figures, then we could cut down cancer rates dramatically. However, the emphasis among cancer researchers is very much on finding a cure rather than reducing the incidence of cancer Since there is so much evidence to show that the causative factors can be controlled (cigarettes cause one-third of all cancers in the United Kingdom), that is, to say the least, surprising. There are many explanations for this disastrous misreading of the needs within cancer research. Undoubtedly one important reason is that there are thousands of surgeons, radiologists and radiotherapists (not to mention pure researchers) earning their living from traditional methods of cancer research and control. Public health is not a fashionable speciality within the medical profession: there is no opportunity for private practice and a general lack of financial incentive for brighter physicians to enter this field. And of equal importance perhaps is the fact that industrial pressures all oppose attempts to control the causative factors responsible for the vast majority of cancers. Trade union leaders seem happier to let their members die than to press for greater safety standards. There can be little doubt that if trade unions did put pressure on employers, factories would be much safer places. The union leaders, however, seem well aware of the fact that safe factories are not necessarily highly profitable factories, since the cost of protecting employees can be high. Employers and union representatives alike appear to have settled for higher profits and higher wages rather than fewer industrial casualties. Little money is spent on protecting employees in proven danger but large sums are spent on research projects designed to find cures. This money, often from public funds, does not affect profits or wages.

I doubt if you will even think of all this next time you see a stranger shaking a collecting tin at you and asking for a contribution towards cancer research. You, like everyone else, have been lured over the years into believing the claims and promises made by honestly motivated but misdirected cancer researchers. If you really cared about cancer patients you would give your money to a caring organisation or an antismoking campaign, taking note of Lord Zuckerman's conclusion in his official Report entitled Cancer Research', published in 1972. He wrote that 'a sudden increase in funds for cancer research could not be effectively used' and suggested that money be spent on helping those struggling to look after relatives dying of cancer rather than on more research programmes.

6. Genetics Research

In the past the creature known as Homo sapiens has altered and developed to suit different environmental conditions through the slow process known as evolution. Man has learned to walk erect, has lost his body hair, has learned to use his hands to make tools and has lost the ability to waggle his ears, through the selection process which ensures that important skills remain and useless skills disappear. The caveman who could make clubs to kill prey and enemies survived, whereas the caveman who could waggle his ears but could not make a club would starve to death and fail to breed. In the past it has been the strong and best adapted who have survived; only in our modern society have the weak and poorly adapted stood a chance of surviving to breed.

The strength, skill and intellect of the average man today is a tribute to the natural selection process which has favoured the fit and healthy and able and worked against the weak and incapacitated. Unfortunately, in modern Western society, where the weak and incapacitated are protected, allowed to have families and encouraged to live as normal a life as possible, the natural selection process no longer works. The average man of tomorrow will, if things continue in the present style, be far less strong, skilful and able. Today, through our medical skills, we encourage the survival of genes which would have been self-limiting a few centuries ago.

We now know of over 1,000 diseases which are caused by genetic defects and we are learning each year how to cope with more and more of these diseases. Some, like phenylketonuria, can be controlled by diet; others, like pyloric stenosis, can be controlled by surgery; yet others can be controlled by artificial supplements in the same way that diabetes can be controlled with the aid of insulin. We are at present unselective about treatment methods – anyone who can be cured is cured and allowed to transmit their illness on to another generation.

Consider for example the disorder known as infantile pyloric stenosis in which the top end of the intestinal tract is narrowed. This is a fairly common genetically determined disorder which affects

about 1 in every 500 babies born. In 1920 the mortality of babies
born with the disorder was 90 per cent. In other words 9 out of 10
babies born with pyloric stenosis died at birth, or shortly afterwards.
Today the mortality rate is down to 1 per cent in some centres,
according to Dr Carter, the Director of the Medical Research
Council's Genetics Unit. The result is that, through expensive
surgery involving the skills of many surgeons, these badly deformed
babies are kept alive. These babies then grow up and have children
of their own. There is a greater than usual chance that their children
will also have pyloric stenosis. Its incidence has increased fiftyfold
since the operation for its cure became commonly available. Similar
increases in the frequency of congenital heart malformations and
other congenital disorders will occur as we learn to keep alive those
with genetic problems.

The incidence of spina bifida is roughly the same as that of
pyloric stenosis but here there are additional problems. Only about
20 per cent of babies born with spina bifida would survive without
surgery, but with surgery many of the rest can be saved. They will
live on, not as normal people but as deformed and handicapped
people with alert brains but dependent bodies. They are often
incapable of looking after themselves, let alone of earning a living.
The result is a tremendous continuing load on the medical services,
the educational services, the patient's family and so on. And as more
spina bifida babies survive and have babies of their own, so the
chances are that the incidence of the disease in the community will
grow.

It is difficult for a doctor, or indeed for any human being to
accept the thought that these people should be left to die. All our
natural feelings ensure that we do what we can to help every patient.
We can ignore the fact that many patients will die because we cannot
afford to provide them with the treatment they need, and we can
even ignore the fact that many of the patients we save live miserable
lives in poorly financed institutions, but we cannot accept the fact
that as a matter of policy babies with spina bifida, for example,
should be left to die when born. Any reports of doctors who do not
provide badly deformed babies with all the resources at their
command meet with a disgusted and angry response.

The thinking observer must find this state of affairs worrying. As
we become capable of treating or saving more and more children

with severe genetic problems, so the genetic quality of man will fall, so the number of dependent people needing permanent nursing and medical care will rise and so the strains and pressures on the shrinking number of perfectly fit and healthy people will increase.

Experts in the field of genetics feel, however, that it is most unlikely that the birth frequencies of genetically determined conditions will be allowed to rise substantially as the result of new methods of treatment, although they agree that the incidence of Down's Syndrome *could* double in a few generations. The more optimistic scientists argue that the future is brighter not bleaker. Dr Amitai Etzioni of Columbia University, speaking at an international meeting said that genetic technology has the potential to take human heredity out of the realm of blind fate or chance into the realm of free will and choice.

There are a variety of ways in which we can control the incidence of genetically determined abnormalities. Some scientists have argued that at birth skin or blood samples of every baby could be fed into a computerised genetic scanner which would note and keep a record of any chromosomal abnormalities. Then, when two people applied for a marriage licence, their cards would be scanned. The potential parent carrying deformed chromosomes would not be allowed to have children. Or, in a less totalitarian society, they might simply receive advice.

Others believe that the best and easiest solution is simply to abort deformed foetuses. By a procedure known as *amniocentesis*, which involves taking a small sample of cells from the fluid around the foetus during pregnancy, doctors can make a prenatal diagnosis of any abnormality. They can determine the baby's sex, they can tell whether or not there are any chromosomal abnormalities (such as Down's Syndrome), they can diagnose metabolic disorders and identify malformations such as spina bifida. In some parts of the world wealthy parents are already taking advantage of such facilities to check on the quality of their unborn sons and daughters and to ensure that the baby they have is the right sex. Professor McKeown, a specialist in the subject of social medicine, believes that selective abortion is the only effective method of reducing the incidence of congenital diseases.

Unfortunately, before amniocentesis is performed, the position of the placenta must first be determined by means of a procedure known as ultrasound. This is a procedure which was first used in the detection of U boats. Waves of high frequency sound energy, above the range of the human ear, are bounced back from distant surfaces. The further away the surface they hit, the weaker the returning signal. With the aid of ultrasound expert technicians can draw plans of the uterus, showing where the foetus is and where the placenta is. If ultrasound is not used, the needle with which a sample of the amniotic fluid which bathes the foetus is obtained may puncture the placenta, with fatal results for the foetus, whether it is healthy or deformed.

We do not yet know whether ultrasound or amniocentesis carry any dangers. According to Harry Harris, writing in *Prenatal Diagnosis and Selective Abortion*, published by the Nuffield Provincial Hospitals Trust in 1974, `…it is not yet possible to say whether disturbances in infant development as indicated by the standard milestones or other abnormalities, for example hearing deficits, which might conceivably be a consequence of an early disturbance of the foetus in utero, occur more frequently if amniocentesis is carried out.'

The dangers of ultrasound and of amniocentesis are worrying many doctors. In *The Lancet* in July 1975, G.E. Smythe and D.J. MacRae of the Mothers' Hospital, London E5, wrote a letter entitled `Doppler ultrasound and foetal hazard' in which they referred to reports which showed that ultrasound causes increased foetal activity. This, they suggested, means that ultrasound is powerful enough `to excite an auditory response in the foetus'. The next step in this logical chain is to ask whether or not ultrasound can damage hearing. This is a question to which we will not know the answer for a few years yet. Meanwhile, ultrasound is gaining popularity (there is a journal devoted to the subject) and the machines, which cost about £25,000 each, are still being used to spot multiple pregnancies, to judge foetal growth rate and to map out the area of the placenta so that amniocentesis can be done in relative safety. Amniocentesis, incidentally, is said by one expert from a Birmingham hospital to be so dangerous that when it is done the number of babies spontaneously aborted greatly exceeds the number of deformed foetuses which would be identified.

According to an editorial in the *British Medical Journal* on 29 November 1975 entitled `Risks of amniocentesis', there is sufficient cause for concern about the safety of the technique for its usefulness to be limited for the time being. According to the leader writer, the safety of amniocentesis needs to be improved before the advantages of the information to be gained clearly outweigh the potential disadvantages. The problem is, of course, that in order for us to obtain information about the usefulness of amniocentesis, the technique must be used on some patients.

Another possibility is selective breeding. Farmers and cattle breeders already use this system for ensuring that their stock is healthy. Fertilised ova are taken from good quality cows and put into cows of inferior genetic quality. The recipient cow then carries on with the mundane business of actually producing the calf. According to Rowson in the 1974 Woolridge Memorial Lecture, the advantages of the technique include the fact that it is possible to increase rapidly the number of good quality cattle on a farm and the fact that the incidence of twins can be increased by putting two fertilised ova into the uterus of the recipient cow.

Artificial insemination is a well-tried technique in farming and it is one not unknown in medical practice. Women whose husbands are infertile can purchase sperm from an unknown donor and have the sperm introduced into the womb artificially. Not unnaturally those who supply the sperm ensure that their donors are strong and healthy. Medical students in the United States often open deposit accounts with sperm banks. It is only a matter of time before commercial groups are providing an even more specific service: 'How tall would you like your son to be, Mrs B?'

Some doctors have suggested that the sterilisation of those carrying bad genes might be the answer. It has been suggested that such sterilisation programmes would benefit both the individual and society. However, such proposals have quite rightly attracted a great deal of opposition from those worried about the rights of the people concerned. On 17 September 1975, an historic judgment was made in the High Court in Britain when Mrs Justice Heilbron ordered doctors to abandon their plans to sterilise an 11-year-old girl with a rare congenital disease which meant that she was physically advanced for her age but mentally handicapped.

Doctors had proposed the sterilisation for the girl's sake and the proposal had been supported by some on philosophical grounds. However, the doctors' plans had been opposed by a female educational psychologist who brought the action to stop the operation. Mrs Justice Heilbron commented that the doctors concerned had 'shown too hasty a disregard for advice from other than purely medical sources'. The point was made in a *Daily Telegraph* editorial the following day that 'there are in fact very few medical decisions that can be taken purely on the basis of clinical judgments, and the recognition of this is not the least important part of a doctor's discipline.' A Labour MP Mr Robert Kilroy-Silk was less tactful: he was reported to have said, 'Thank God we have the courts to protect us against the doctors'.

Other doctors have begun to examine the possibilities of genetic surgery, of developing the ability to take out undesirable genes, and replace them with others which will ensure that the next generation will be fit and bright. We could in theory breed all men or all women, or breed men as we breed race horses, favouring those genes which provide the qualities we think are important. In the more immediate future we could use genetic surgery to help ensure that all babies born were relatively healthy and likely to develop into physically and mentally healthy adults.

When historians look at the end of this century and try to pick out the most important medical achievement, the single most devastating advance, they may well choose not the first heart transplant operation or the introduction of penicillin but the development of the various techniques for growing and studying human cells in the laboratory – breeding what are popularly known as test-tube babies. Doing this enables us to diagnose genetic deformities at an early stage and to operate on genes likely to produce abnormalities.

The nucleus in an egg contains half of the number of chromosomes which will be contained in the cells of the fully grown animal. Scientists have already shown that if they take the nucleus from a frog's egg before fertilisation and then replace that nucleus with the nucleus from an ordinary cell, the egg will develop into a frog which has the same characteristics as the frog from which the cell was taken.

What this means is that if a man and woman plan to have a family but find out that the woman carries genes which are likely to result in their child being deformed, they can seek help from a scientist who will remove the nucleus from one of the woman's eggs and replace it with the nucleus from a physically perfect and intelligent woman's egg which does not carry genes likely to produce a deformed child. This egg with its new nucleus will then be fertilised by sperm from the husband and it can either be nurtured in the laboratory or it can be put back into the woman's womb for her to nurture it herself.

When the resultant baby is born it will carry the inherited characteristics of the father and the woman who donated the egg nucleus. It is not difficult to see from this that it would in theory be quite possible to breed millions of people who were all pretty similar simply by putting the nuclei from one woman's cells into the eggs of other women. The world could then be filled with millions of women looking like Sophia Loren.

By cross fertilisation between species it might also be possible to breed people who have the advantages of other species. For example, we could perhaps breed people able to regenerate missing limbs as newts do. It may be possible to breed human females who lay eggs rather than have babies; we may be able to breed smaller human beings so that more of us can crowd on to our small planet; we may be able to breed legless men to take jobs as astronauts (a spaceman has no need for legs) and we may even be able to breed men and women with chlorophyll beneath their skin so that they can photosynthesise themselves, turning useless carbon dioxide into life-giving oxygen. Perhaps we will be able to encourage the body to accept foreign implants. There are endless possibilities. A woman who produces no eggs at all and who cannot therefore have children of her own could borrow an egg cell from another woman, remove its nucleus and replace it with one of her own before having the egg cell placed in her own uterus for fertilisation by her husband. The sperm cell would then combine with the egg cell and the woman and husband would give birth to a child of their own.

There are, however, as many dangers as there are possibilities in genetic research. Researchers studying genes have for some time been using bacteria for their basic studies because the genetic systems of bacteria are relatively simple. There is also the added advantage that bacteria reproduce in minutes rather than in weeks or months so that long-term studies can more easily be carried out. The bacterium most commonly used is one called Escherichia Coli, a bug found in the human gut. The researchers change the genetic information carried by each bacterium by cross breeding, by chemical treatments and even by genetic surgery, using enzymes as tools with which to chop up chromosomes. According to a World Health Organisation statement on the subject, The innovative techniques of DNA recombination consist in isolating and then splicing together DNA molecules from unrelated organisms to produce a new hybrid organism which may contain the genetic properties of either or both or the original organisms. Researchers are also already experimenting with the fusion of cells and the growth in culture of cells containing nuclei from completely different sources.

With these experiments research biologists hope to gain an understanding of the way in which genes are controlled and the way they work to produce healthy or diseased tissues and organs. Researchers hope to be able eventually to develop ways of manufacturing vital substances. For example, if the segments of DNA which are responsible for the production of insulin can be introduced into the E.coli organism, the bacteria culture would act as a factory producing insulin.

Research workers have already learnt how to transfer antibiotic resistance from one bacterium to another. They use this technique to help them mark particular genes as effectively as if they had initialled them. Unfortunately, the manufacture of resistant organisms is potentially very dangerous for it would theoretically be possible for resistant organisms to get out of the laboratory and into the community. These organisms could then cause infections in innocent people and doctors would be unable to treat the infections because the organisms responsible were resistant to available drugs.

There are other dangers involved. It is, for example, particularly dangerous to experiment with a bacterium such as E.coli, a common inhabitant of the human gastro-intestinal tract, because if by accident a lethal version of E.coli got out of the laboratory, it would be able to kill off millions of people quite easily. Genetic information such as that carried in viruses which cause tumours might be introduced into E.coli, and when the newly knowledgeable E.coli found itself inside a human being it would be able to start a tumour.

Even the researchers themselves admit that almost anything is possible in the field of genetics and that we just do not know enough to tell whether a particular piece of research is potentially dangerous or not.

Of course, researchers do take precautions. They wear masks and keep the doors and windows closed when experimenting with dangerous or potentially dangerous organisms, but such traditional precautions are hardly likely to prove effective it a really dangerous bacterium is produced. And, of course, laboratories searching for weapons (whether financed by governments or by industry) will deliberately try to produce lethal bacteria. There is, in particular, the danger of human error. It was, after all, carelessness in a laboratory which led to an outbreak of smallpox in London in 1973, resulting in several deaths and costing several million pounds to contain.

Worried by these many possibilities and various dangers some scientists have already called for a halt. In May 1972 the *Journal of the American Medical Association* called, without much success, for a moratorium on attempts to implant into a woman's womb an ovum fertilised outside the body. In July 1974 eleven leading molecular biologists working in America had a letter published in *Science* in which they publicly stated their fears about two particular types of experiments involving the use of genes.

One of the scientists who signed the letter, Paul Berg of the University of Stamford, California, was one of the first men to discover the enzymes with which genes can be taken apart and put back together. These enzymes are the equivalents of the surgeon's tools. Berg and his colleagues were particularly worried that the research they described could result in the development of dangerous organisms, especially organisms resistant to known methods of treatment. Sir John Kendrew, President of the British Association, told the Association's annual meeting in Stirling that the bacterium most commonly used in genetic research could inadvertently be given a cancer gene which might spread cancer in humans. Sir John, who is Deputy Chairman of the MC's Laboratory of Molecular Biology, said that the problems could be greater than those raised by the atomic bomb.

One result of the controversy over the dangers of genetic research was that in Britain a `Working Party on the Experimental Manipulation of the Genetic Composition of Microorganisms' was set up under Lord Ashby. It included thirteen members of whom only three seemed to be doctors. None of these were in active practice. The other members of the Working Party included the director of a poultry research station, the director of a plant breeding institute at Cambridge and the Secretary of the Agricultural Research Council. The Working Party was appointed to `assess the potential benefits and potential hazards of techniques which allow the experimental manipulation of the genetic composition of micro-organisms'.

Naturally, a committee made up largely of specialist workers in the field under inquiry could hardly be expected to see the potential problems in their true light. Like warriors with bows and arrows who assume that their shields will protect them against any weapon they come up against, the members of the Working Party assumed that any potential hazards could be prevented or at least minimised by currently available techniques. They completely ignored the fact that researchers are moving into new territory where they do not know what will happen. They also ignored the problems of human error, commercial greed, mental illness and psychopathic workers. They assumed that all workers in this field are quite perfect.

They admitted that many bacterial geneticists and molecular biologists are unfamiliar with the hazards involved and the precautions needed; they agreed that the techniques of genetic manipulation are comparatively easy to master and cheap to perform but refused to insist on minimal operating precautions.

The Working Party reported to the Government in January 1975 that 'research into genetic engineering should be allowed to continue because the potential benefits to medicine outweigh the dangers which can be safeguarded against'. Opponents of the suggested moratorium had argued that the work had such enormous individual and military potential that it would be impossible to stop and that it would therefore be unfair to close down Government-sponsored laboratories.

In June 1975 the Advisory Committee on Medical Research of the WHO also discussed at length the safety problems involved in the experimental handling of pathogenic organisms. This committee, also mainly composed of research workers, similarly decided that most hazards could be kept under control voluntarily by techniques already in use and implied that there were no additional risks.

All the research I have described is therefore still continuing. Progress is fairly fast in this particular field and many of the things I have outlined have already been done.

7. Transplant Research

Artificial legs have been used as replacements for missing lower limbs since the year 600 BC, and metal hands have been provided for unfortunate patients since the sixteenth century. However, it has been during the last few decades that the greatest advances in organ replacement have been made. Of the vital internal organs, it was the kidneys which first became replaceable.

The kidneys have the important task of regulating electrolyte and water content in the body. They also help to eliminate potentially harmful waste products which result from food metabolism. People whose kidneys fail or are destroyed or damaged will die a slow but certain death if they are not provided with some form of alternative kidney to do the work of their own ineffective organs. The human body can manage quite well on one kidney, so it is only when both are badly damaged that the danger arises. Unhappily there are thousands of people each year who do die through kidney diseases. Some have had high blood pressure which has destroyed the kidneys, some have had tumours which have destroyed the active kidney tissue, but most have simply had bad infections which have rendered the kidneys *hors de combat*.

The first artificial kidney was developed by a Dutch surgeon, Dr Willem J. Kolff, working 'underground' during the German occupation of his country in the Second World War. He developed a machine which sent blood flowing outside the body through a cellophane container which was submerged in a solution of salt and glucose. Cellophane is a semi-permeable barrier and the unwanted blood contents passed out through this barrier into the solution of salt and glucose. The blood left the cellophane container and was ready to pick up more impurities via the kidneys again. At the same time as the waste products left the blood, salt and glucose entered it. To make sure that the blood did not clot in the cellophane tube Dr Kolff added an anti-coagulant, a substance which interferes with the normal clotting mechanism of the blood.

Modern artificial kidneys are merely improved versions of this simple machine. One important improvement was added by Dr Kolff himself when in 1956 he produced a disposable cellophane container.

The original artificial kidney had a number of disadvantages. The patient had to be connected to it at least once a week to have his blood cleaned out and different blood vessels had to be used each time. For the blood to leave the body and pass through the cellophane kidney', it had to be taken out from one blood vessel and returned via another. Inevitably that meant that after a while patients ran out of usable blood vessels. There were none left to which the machine could be connected. Even in those early days, however, there were too many patients for the number of machines available and doctors had to take the painful decision of who was to benefit from treatment and who was to be left to die. In some areas committees were set up with the idea of helping doctors decide whom to save.

In the early 1960s doctors at the University of Washington School of Medicine in Seattle designed a valve which could be left permanently in place in the body. Made of rubber and plastic (which would not excite a rejection reaction in the body) the valve is U shaped. Normally it sits comfortably in the patient's body allowing blood to flow into it from a vein and out of it into an artery. When the patient needs to be dialysed he can simply plug the artificial kidney into his valve.

Today's artificial kidneys can be used with comparative ease, often by the patient himself at home. The only problem, of course, is the cost. It is difficult to give figures since costs vary depending upon the amount of skilled help required but it certainly costs several thousand pounds a year to keep a patient alive on an artificial kidney and we can still only afford to save a very small proportion of those who need artificial dialysis.

The alternative to kidney dialysis or the artificial kidney is a kidney transplant. Here the theory is simple: a good, working kidney is taken from someone else and put into the patient whose kidneys do not work. The kidney donor may be a close relative who chooses to donate a kidney to save a life, or a complete stranger who died suddenly, usually in a road accident, and who had one or two perfectly healthy kidneys. When a relative wishes to give a patient a kidney, twin operations are performed in adjoining operating theatres. The kidney to be donated is removed by one surgeon in one theatre and placed in the patient by another surgeon in the other theatre. The advantage with this type of operation is that the kidney will be more likely to fit into the patient's body without being rejected as `foreign' and it will therefore have a much greater chance of lasting and working properly. Just as close relatives sometimes share facial characteristics, so their internal organs share certain tissue characteristics.

A kidney from a dead patient must be taken almost immediately and it must be stored properly if it is to be usable. Doctors try to make sure that the kidneys they put into patients are acceptable and will not be rejected. They do this by examining the tissues of the recipient and the donor and checking that they are compatible. It is rather like making sure that blood being given to a patient comes from a donor with the right blood group. Sometimes a kidney will be taken from a dead patient in one hospital and put into a living patient in another hospital. Then, of course, there will be a dramatic dash between the two hospitals with the kidney carefully packed in a special container. Again there are nowhere near enough surgeons, surgical teams and donor kidneys available to provide all patients who need one with a kidney transplant.

In the summer of 1975 Sir Henry Yellowlees, Chief Medical Officer at the Department of Health and Social Security, pointed out that 900 patients with chronic renal failure were waiting for suitable transplant kidneys in the United Kingdom alone. Another 600 patients are added to this list each year and those patients who have had transplants often return for a second transplant kidney a year or two later.

Donors are in great demand. Figures in Britain suggest that less than 10 per cent of all dying people in hospital are likely to be suitable kidney donors. A report in the *Journal of the American Medical Association* in 1975 showed that only a quarter of the people suggested as possible donors turned out to be suitable. The result of the shortage of donors in one area of America was that of 642 patients waiting for a transplant, only 175 received one. Australian doctors, anxious to do more for patients with renal failure, have started to prepare possible donors for transplantation before death. People considered likely to have usable kidneys are given special treatment while they are still alive to ensure that their kidneys remain usable. Other doctors believe, however, that it is ethically wrong to regard a patient as merely a potential donor and to treat him as such.

Most of the kidneys which are transplanted are taken from corpses – or cadavers, as dead bodies are technically known – and according to the *Drug and Therapeutic Bulletin* in October 1975, 30 per cent of the patients who are given kidneys taken from cadavers are in trouble within two years. These patients either die or need new transplants.

An important cause of death in most 'developed' countries is heart disease. There are many ways in which a heart can go wrong. It may start beating irregularly; it may develop a clot which kills off part of the actual heart tissue; it may simply fail to function properly. The techniques used to solve the problem depend, of course, upon the problem itself.

The heart beats because of electrical impulses which pass through the heart muscle from a point in the right atrium. Normally these electrical impulses set off about 70 beats a minute. Occasionally however, the impulses are irregular and the heart does not beat properly. In these cases the patient can sometimes be helped if a device known as a 'pacemaker' is implanted.

It was in 1950 that electric shock treatments were first used to stimulate the heart. The machine known as a defibrillator is simply a rather fancy contraption for giving electric shocks to patients. It is used when a patient in hospital has a sudden heart attack which results in the cessation of the heartbeat. The aim is for the electrical shock to restart the heart. Sometimes it works. The defibrillator probably helps the coronary care unit to save the lives of some patients who have severe heart attacks while in the unit.

The defibrillator is, however, a bulky instrument which usually travels about on a small trolley. It would be most impractical for a patient to carry one about with him. For this reason in the late 1950s doctors started fitting smaller pacemakers to some of their patients. The pacemakers simply gave small electric shocks directly to the heart, taking over the job of the faulty source in the right atrium. The original pacemakers were powered by batteries which had to be replaced every couple of years but some patients are now being fitted with atomic pacemakers.

Some patients have hearts which beat regularly but which do not function properly because of valvular disease. Inside the heart there are four valves which allow the flow of blood through in one direction only and which stop the back flow of blood. Sometimes these valves fail to function with the result that blood does not flow through properly. The heart then does not work correctly and the patient will develop symptoms of some kind of heart failure. Surgeons can now perform operations to repair or replace these faulty valves; the repairs usually involve the installation of specially designed plastic valves.

Other patients have hearts which do not work properly because a blood clot has stopped the correct flow of blood to the heart muscle. In these cases surgeons can help either by cleaning out the blocked blood vessels (rather as the plumber clears out blocked pipes) or by replacing totally blocked pipes with new ones. Sometimes a small length of vein taken from another part of the patient's own body can be used to replace the diseased tube.

Many patients do, of course, have hearts which are too badly damaged to respond to fresh and regular electrical stimulation. If these patients are to survive, they need new hearts. A few years ago this would have seemed totally impossible. However, we now know that it can be done.

The first animal-to-animal heart transplantation operation was performed as long ago as 1905, although it was not until 1964 that two workers at Stamford University in California wrote that 'cardiac homograft's are just around the corner.' In that same year a surgeon at the University of Mississippi transplanted a chimpanzee heart into a human patient, and in 1968 a surgeon finally transplanted a human heart from one patient to another. That was the beginning of many such operations.

This first heart transplant was done in South Africa by Dr Christiaan Barnard. In other parts of that country the WHO estimates that there are one million black children suffering from malnutrition and that babies have only a 50 per cent chance of reaching the age of 5 years. Roy Calne, an eminent British surgeon and academic, has said, 'To argue that money could be better spent in preventive medicine or underdeveloped countries is irrelevant.' Transplant surgeons are a race apart. They are extraordinarily fond of the limelight (remember the British Transplant Team with their Union Jacks and beaming smiles?) and apparently uninterested in the larger problems they create. Those who think this assessment harsh should remember that those unfortunate patients who were in the right place at the right time to suffer the unnecessary pain involved in having a heart transplanted were doomed from the start – and observers knew it. Every doctor knew that if those hearts were not to be rejected by the other tissues, the patient would have to have his rejection mechanisms neutralised and that if this were done he could be killed by the first infection to attack him, since the mechanisms which reject strange hearts are the same as those which attack and reject strange germs.

The problems with transplanting hearts are similar to those which confront surgeons transplanting kidneys. There is a shortage of suitable donors since the donor must have a healthy heart and must die quite suddenly and certainly within reach of a heart transplant centre. And the surgeon has the additional problem of finding a donor with a heart which will fit into the needy patient's body without inspiring a rejection problem. The difficulties have not yet been solved. Indeed, according to the *Drug and Therapeutics Bulletin* for 10 October 1975, `the kidney is the only organ which can be transplanted at all reliably'.

For those patients with badly diseased hearts the only possible alternative to a heart transplantation is the implantation of an artificial heart. Since several million people die every year from heart failure, there would clearly be a tremendous market for an implantable artificial heart. The surgeon who first put an artificial heart into a patient was Dr Denton Cooley of Houston. The operation was performed in 1969 and Cooley was accused by some of pirating the heart from a research effort headed by another Houston heart surgeon, Dr Michael E. DeBakey.

Since then a number of surgeons, engineers, cardiologists, physicists and industrial experts have been busy searching for the correct design. Dr Kolff, the man who invented the first artificial kidney put together a team of workers to set about the problem. He is quoted as saying that 600,000 people a year could be helped with an artificial heart.

The problems involved in designing an artificial heart are enormous. A pump has to be designed that can move several pints of blood every minute and never rest. It must build up just the right amount of pressure and distribute fresh blood to the body and exhausted blood to the lungs. Those working with artificial hearts do at least have the advantage that they do not have to snatch their replacement hearts from dead and dying patients. When effective artificial hearts are available, as they will be shortly, the main problem will be a financial one. The cost of installing an artificial heart is equivalent to the cost of purchasing a large house.

Transplant surgeons have not ignored other internal organs. Lung and liver transplants have been tried without much success and work is in progress to try and develop artificial replacements for almost all faulty organs. An artificial gut has already been built which can help patients who have damaged or diseased intestines. Skin banks have been in existence for some time and plastic surgeons use them to help repair badly burnt patients. Artificial skin is proving difficult to produce, mainly because the skin is always regenerating and scientists are encountering problems in creating a self-regenerating type of skin.

Surgeons now also use elastic, seamless, corrugated, almost indestructible dacron arteries to replace diseased blood vessels, steel bones and joints to replace arthritic and damaged parts, silicon breasts to supplement or replace natural glands, electric pacemakers to stimulate weary hearts, and will soon be using artificial hearts, kidneys and lungs to replace damaged organs physically, as well as treating burns with plastic skin. According to the British Medical Association, total hip replacement is now almost a major industry in this country. The surgical instrument makers Down Brothers sell hips, knees, elbows, finger joints and big toes in their catalogue. As Dr Richard Gordon, writing: in the *Daily Telegraph* Magazine, put it, 'Frankenstein's monster is alive, if not very well, and living unnoticed in the instrument makers' catalogues.'

A Japanese surgeon recently designed and fitted a titanium and polythene thigh bone that can be accurately fitted to the patient when it is installed. Other orthopaedic surgeons use cords of woven dacron to repair or replace damaged tendons. One American patient went back to competitive wrestling eight weeks after a surgeon had repaired his damaged shoulder with dacron tubing. Cardiac surgeons have for two decades been replacing damaged heart valves; in America Cooley has himself implanted some 4,300 heart valves while DeBakey has implanted over 3,000.

Development in all areas of transplantation and replacement is rapid. Surgeons fixing artificial limbs will in the near future link the prosthesis directly to the patient's nervous system to enable the amputee to manipulate his artificial limb merely by willing a particular movement. It has even been suggested that patients will in the not too distant future have planned amputations of perfectly healthy limbs so that they can replace these limbs with a selection of limb extensions designed like mechanical tools. Thomas Edison wrote that The body is just something to carry the brain around in' and as artificial limbs become stronger, more reliable and more inventive, so people will be more and more interested in replacing their own limbs with something better.

Tomorrow's hospital may well, it seems, have to include a 'spare parts' department on each complex. Though the prospect is undoubtedly attractive to those who are unable to accept the fact that man is a mortal being, there will be many problems. The fact that transplants merely provide temporary and expensive solutions for a small number of individual problems, the ethical rows which have developed over the use of organs from still-living patients, and the horrifying cost of each operation led the Chief Medical Officer of the Department of Health and Social Security to decree that we in Britain should not waste money and effort on heart transplant attempts until more reliable and economical methods have been evolved.

Transplants and artificial organs certainly offer hope to some patients, who would otherwise he let without any hope at all. Whether the hope is justified depends on the type of replacement. (A hip replacement is much more justifiable than a heart replacement – it will work.) But in the long term transplantation can offer only a pseudo-solution. Developing artificial hearts and artificial kidneys may offer something to those already suffering but will do nothing to prevent future patients developing exactly the same problem. The transplanted organ provides symptomatic relief at great cost both to the recipient and to the community. It will never be possible for us to provide replacement organs for all those who need them. But it might well be possible to prevent the need for replacement organs from arising in a large proportion of patients.

Not content with merely attempting to replace parts of the human body which have failed to function properly, researchers are now also working on ways of improving the human body by adding to it. Steve Austin, the hero of the television series *Six Million Dollar*

Man, is supposed to have lost both legs, one arm and an eye in a space-ship crash. These missing parts have been replaced with bionic items giving Austin superhuman qualities which enable him to run at 60 mph, leap high fences, spot villains in the dim distance, fight with the strength of ten men and generally act the part of superman. Unlike many such television programmes, *Six Million Dollar Man* does not exaggerate the possibilities. The title, incidentally, refers, quite realistically, to the estimated cost of such an operation.

The first developments in this field involved the use of arm or leg extensions. One system, for example, involves a man crouching inside a 3,000-pound metal monster. The man is effectively the monster's brain. He is electronically linked to the limbs, and the design of the system amplifies and exaggerates his every movement. If, for instance, the man inside the monster wishes to move a railway sleeper out of his way he merely has to flick his wrist in the correct direction. The movement is magnified and given extra strength. This monster was developed for the American Army.

Ophthalmic surgeons are currently developing artificial eyes made like small television cameras which fit into the eye sockets and transmit signals direct to the visual cortex. When these cameras are fitted with zoom lenses (as they undoubtedly will be), the handicapped person will have an advantage over the fit and normal person. Sportsmen, ambitious workers and those with military responsibilities will obviously be more than willing to have unnecessary surgery and improve their own abilities.

Researchers have now shown that every single gesture and indeed every single thought involves a measurable electrical potential and can therefore be used to operate machinery. Already in existence are experimental automobile braking systems which can be activated merely by lifting an eyebrow, and guns linked to the human eye which fire at whatever the eye is focused on, using as a trigger a firm flick of the eye.

According to *Time* magazine for 1 December 1975, a 24-year-old Californian karate expert, Reid Hilton, who lost his right arm in an accident now has a 40,000-dollar replacement myoelectric arm 'developed at Northwestern University and modified by engineers and researchers at the Medical Products Division of General Atomic and at Ranchos Los Amigos, a hospital associated with the University of California'. Hilton's arm has a power pack in the prosthesis, is fitted with feedback devices which give a sense of touch and is directly connected to nerves in the stump of his severed arm. A normal male grip exerts a force of about 25 pounds but Hilton's electronically assisted grip strength is an impressive 40 pounds.

The day of the mechanical man is not far away.

8. Working on the Mind

One-third of all the patients seen by general practitioners are said to have mental problems of one sort or another. It has been shown that 20 per cent of students at British universities suffer from some form of mental disorder at some stage in their university course. Only 35 per cent of a rural French population were free of psychiatric disorders, according to another study. In. Paris some 25 per cent of all cases of incapacity for work were caused by mental illness and in a Canadian study of 400,000 people only 20 per cent showed no mental disturbances. Most of these figures appear in a book entitled *Health in 1980-90. A predictive study based on an international inquiry* by Philip Selby which was sponsored by a drug company together with the Henry Dunant Institute of the Red Cross, and they give us a pretty good idea of what is likely to be the major medical problem of the future.

Medical researchers have, naturally, spent a good deal of effort on investigating possible cures for mental problems. The cures they have studied fall into several distinct groups. Firstly there are the pharmacological cures. Most of the major drug companies are already involved in the search for drugs to alleviate anxiety and depression and the number of drugs already on the market is growing at an astonishing rate. Most of the new drugs which, come out are said to be specific for particular types of psychological problem – for example, for phobic anxiety. Many researchers in this field are confident that within a few years they will be able to control most human emotions with the aid of specific drugs, although they admit that they must first come to a more complete understanding of biochemical and electrical pathways within the brain.

Though few researchers are modest enough to admit it, acquiring a total understanding of the way the brain works is likely to be a slow business. The brain contains three times as many cells as there are human beings on the earth and these cells are interconnected by a series of electronic and biochemical pathways which make even the most sophisticated modern computer look like an abacus. Since many of the computers we are making today are almost beyond our comprehension, the chances of anyone understanding the workings of the human brain must be that much less. In addition, there are philosophical problems, for some believe that it is quite impossible for the human brain ever to completely understand itself. The more you think about it the more perplexing this particular problem seems to be.

The next and probably so far most controversial area of brain control is brain surgery. Some brain surgery is, of course, lifesaving. There is, however, much brain surgery which is of less value; in particular I am referring to prefrontal leucotomy in which a part of the brain is permanently and deliberately damaged.

The first leucotomies were performed in the 1930s when it was thought that the frontal lobes were the source of delusions in mental patients. American workers removed the frontal lobes of chimpanzees in 1935 and thought that their animals were more contented afterwards. In the following year a neurosurgeon working in Portugal tested the theory, and injected alcohol into the frontal lobes of 20 schizophrenics.

Then, until the 1950s, thousands of patients had surgical operations to cut off their frontal lobes. Today such surgery is still performed frequently though there is no proper evidence to show that it does any good at all. Since those who have had the operation are rather quiet, apparently dim and contented people, few of them have complained.

Egas Moniz, when Professor of Neurology in Lisbon, was the first to develop leucotomy, though Walter Freeman, then Professor of Neurology at Washington University, took a great interest in the operation. During the ten years from 1940 to 1950 Freeman wrote 56 articles, most of them concerned with neurosurgery. The total number of papers written on the subject runs into thousands. In 1961 it was reported that about 500 operations a year were being performed in the United Kingdom and in 1970 according to Ashley Robin and Duncan Macdonald in *Lessons of Leucotomy*, one surgeon reported that he himself had performed over a thousand operations during the previous ten years. In 1972 it was estimated by Breggin in `Congressional Record' that 50,000 operations had been performed in America and that Freeman had done 4,000 of these. In the *British Medical Journal* of 1971, it was estimated that 100,000 operations had been performed around the world.

Robin and Macdonald, in their careful study of the literature on leucotomy, assessed the reports in existence and concluded that 'Other methods of treatment e.g. tranquillising drugs, were as effective in improving non-operated patients as leucotomy.' They also reported that 'Neither patients with schizophrenia nor depression have a better prospect of discharge after leucotomy. The results in severely phobic and obsessional patients are inconclusive.'

The popularity of psychosurgery in the 1960s was well described in a text book entitled *An introduction to Physical Methods of Treatment in Psychiatry* by Dr William Sargant, Physician in charge of the Department of Psychological Medicine and Lecturer in the St Thomas's Hospital Medical School, London, Dr Eliot Slater, Physician in Psychological Medicine at the National Hospital in Queen Square and Honorary Physician at the Maudsley Hospital, London, and Dr Peter Dally, Physician in Psychological Medicine at the Westminster Hospital, London. I list the authors' qualifications to illustrate their eminence in the medical profession. The book was published by a well-respected company, E. & S. Livingstone Ltd, the fourth edition being dated 1963. According to the authors, over 15,000 leucotomies had been performed in Great Britain by 1963. The operation, involving the cutting away or simply the deliberate damaging of part of the brain, was performed on patients with schizophrenia, depression, obsessional neurosis, anxiety states, hysteria, eczema, asthma, chronic rheumatism, anorexia nervosa, ulcerative colitis, tuberculosis, hypertension, angina and intractable pain due to carcinoma. Leucotomies had even been performed on patients suffering from anxiety caused by barbiturate toxicity.

The operation is described with great enthusiasm in the book with such statements as 'It is probable that nearly every individual after operation is happier than before…', though to be fair some of the problems are also described. It is, for example, admitted that, 'The more subtle powers of the intellect, such as its intuitive and imaginative qualities, may sometimes be affected detrimentally.' The book lists complications such as bedwetting, somnolence, severe and prolonged confusion and paralysis, and the mortality rate is given as I per cent or less, though in a text published ten years later (*Psychiatry* by Anderson and Trethowan) the mortality rate is quoted as nearer to 3 per cent.

Sargant and his fellow writers also warn that a patient may develop epilepsy after the operation and that there may be damage to his personality.

All these dangers and problems are described in subjective fashion, probably because, in 1963, there was little scientific evidence on which to base any proper judgment, and it seems that these three physicians had a great regard for the operation's value. Their faulty judgment can be excused but what is more difficult to excuse is the fact that, without any real and convincing evidence based on the results of properly organised and reported clinical trials, they recommended patients to have an operation which carried enormous risks and indeed involved the destruction of a part of the brain. Without proper trials it could not have been possible to be certain that any improvement noticed was not simply due to the fact that the patients concerned no longer had the capacity to notice their problems. The patient who is lying stupid and senseless in bed is unlikely to complain of his eczema, just as the patient who has died during an operation intended to provide him with a new heart is unlikely to complain of the symptoms of heart failure which had troubled him previously. Living euthanasia is not a treatment which any doctor worthy of the name can recommend today. It is a black mark in the history of medicine that it was ever recommended. It is even more depressing to have to report that it is still being done.

Since most psychosurgery is based on the results of surgery done on a few irritable chimpanzees many years ago, some doctors wonder why more trials have not been done by those who believe in its value. After all, there are plenty more neurotic and psychotic chimpanzees around who could have operations. As an editorial writer in 'The Lancet' put it in May 1975, 'A common attitude to psychosurgery, the neurosurgical approach to the treatment of functional mental illness, is scepticism. This writer estimated that between 200 and 300 neurosurgical operations are done in Britain each year.

In July 1975 it was announced in 'The Lancet' that at long last, a properly organised, controlled trial of psychosurgery was to be set up by the Royal College of Psychiatrists. The idea of the trial was to perform operations on 200 patients with severe mental disease who had failed to respond to conventional therapy. Unfortunately, the trial was heavily criticised by many experts. In the autumn of 1975, the College was still receiving many critical comments from observers who wanted to know how patients would be chosen, who would decide whether or not a particular patient was eligible and how anyone ill enough to need the operation could give consent for it to be done.

The risks of psychosurgery are great and the rewards unproven, so it is difficult to see how controlled clinical trials could ever be undertaken without the use of 'human guinea pigs'. Many doctors (and the number is increasing annually) believe that a psychiatrist who wrote to the `British Medical Journal' in June 1973 had summed up the situation accurately: he argued that performing surgery on a delicate organ like the brain is rather like kicking a television set which doesn't work in the hope that a good kick will make it function normally again. Indeed, psychosurgery is even more illogical – it could perhaps better be compared to simply ripping out some of the insides of a television set to try to make it work.

According to a book entitled `Protection of Human Rights in the light of Scientific and Technological Progress in Biology and Medicine' published by the World Health Organisation in 1974, after a round-table conference of the Council for International Organisations of Medical Sciences, "The procedures in contemporary psychosurgery are based on inadequate or limited research and they entail many hazards. Psychosurgery has unpredictable effects on a precious organ, which, even when a locus of society's discontent, should rarely need a lesion instead of special care.'

The operation of pre-frontal leucotomy is a frightening example of an experimental procedure which has become an accepted part of medical practice without ever having been properly tested. Many papers have been written on the subject but the authors have invariably been practising neurosurgeons, reporting on uncontrolled trials.

The situation today is that the operation is still being performed by a small number of surgeons who refuse to accept that it is an invalid and unethical procedure. Meanwhile, the great majority of practising physicians believe that the operation is so worthless and dangerous that it would be unethical to perform a controlled clinical trial now. They believe that the operation should simply be abandoned and forgotten, to take its place in history with the other fantasy treatments such as blood-letting, and the removal of the intestines for constipation.

The result is an impasse. Those who doubt the operation's value will not involve themselves in trials. Those who do not doubt the operation's value will not involve themselves in trials. And so every year several hundred patients undergo leucotomies at the hands of the obstinate few.

While psychosurgery seems to offer only a crude method of controlling the brain, there are other more subtle methods of control currently being researched. The method with perhaps the most promise (if that is the right word) is the electronic stimulation of the brain. This system depends upon the mapping out of the brain and the identification of the sites within it where various categories of thought and emotion originate. To that extent electronic stimulation of the brain involves the same basic research as psychosurgery. There, however, the similarity ends. Instead of simply destroying part of the brain as the neurosurgeon does when performing psychosurgery, the researcher experimenting with electronic stimulation limits himself to trying to control parts of the brain.

For over a century doctors have known that if wires are poked into the brain and an electric charge passed through them, there will be different responses from different parts of the brain. A wire poked into one part will cause a leg to move, the same wire poked into another part of the brain will give the patient an erection. Today we know that with the aid of electronic stimulation, doctors can induce pleasure, eradicate pain and recall memories previously lost.

In order to put electrodes into the human brain a number of procedures must first be carried out. First, special X-rays are taken, using air (injected into the spaces inside the brain) to enable the doctors to get a real view of the brain's actual shape. Eventually the researchers can tell where to put their electrodes.

Next, small holes are drilled in the skull and hair-thin electrodes are sunk into the brain to the depth the experimenting surgeon desires. The brain has no sense of pain and so the actual insertion of the electrodes into the brain is painless. When the electrodes have been put into position, the exposed ends are fitted with terminals which are fixed to the scalp. To stimulate the brain small amounts of electrical current are passed along the electrodes. Doctors have now developed their techniques to such an extent that they fit small receivers onto the scalp so that electrical impulses can be fired into the brain from afar. The receivers fit under wigs or hats and are supplied with long-lasting batteries. Eventually, no doubt, receivers will be designed which can be fitted under the scalp.

With the electrodes in position the patient can be controlled quite effectively from a distance. He can be made to eat, to sleep or to work. His appetite, heart rate, body temperature and other factors can also be controlled. The system has great possibilities for helping obese patients to slim. It has also been said that it can be used to help the blind to see. Many wired-up patients have proved to have 'pleasure centres' which can be stimulated quite easily. Researchers have noted that patients stimulated in their right places suddenly start talking about sex or acting in a sexually flirtatious manner.

One doctor has predicted that in a not too distant future patients requiring anaesthesia will be taken to the operating theatre fully conscious and put to sleep with the aid of a current sent down an electrode into the brain. Another doctor has reported that he already has epileptic patients who are fitted with electrodes and transmitters of their own. When these patients feel a fit starting they simply press a button and abort the fit.

Researchers have shown that gentle cats can be transformed into aggressive beasts if certain parts of their brains are stimulated. In the 1950s Dr Delgado of the Yale University School of Medicine showed that two cats, normally quite friendly, could be made to fight fiercely if electrodes implanted in the brain were given impulses. Even when it continually lost its fights, the smaller of the two cats continued to be aggressive when stimulated. In one dramatic experiment Dr Delgado wired a bull with electrodes and then planted himself in the middle of a bullring with a cape and a small radio transmitter. The bull charged but was stopped by Dr Delgado pressing a button on his transmitter. The bull screeched to a halt inches away from its target. Dr Delgado has reported that 'Animals with implanted electrodes in their brains have been made to perform a variety of responses with predictable reliability as if they were electronic toys under human control.'

Similar experiments have been performed with human beings. The patients selected had all proved dangerous and had shown that they had uncontrollable tempers. By electronic stimulation every patient was controlled. More detailed accounts of these experiments can be read in *Physical Control of the Mind* by J.M.R. Delgado.

There are now so many neurosurgeons doing operations on the mentally ill (in some parts of America it is said, not entirely jokingly, that it is dangerous to complain of a headache) that other doctors are beginning to worry. There are many instances of patients who have had such surgery becoming worse afterwards; there are reported cases of patients who have had only exploratory operations improving just as much as patients who have destructive surgery; there are also worrying instances of neurosurgeons who have operated on children described as nuisances.

There will always be people who ignore ethical codes. There was a surgeon in the last century in England who achieved great fame by removing several thousand yards of intestine from patients complaining of constipation. These patients developed diarrhoea and lived miserable lives but Arbuthnot Lane, the surgeon, did well out of his work. In October 1899 the medical officer of the Jeffersonville Reformatory in Indiana performed a vasectomy on a patient who was unduly worried about his masturbatory habits. Dr Harry C. Sharp later claimed that the operation of vasectomy made males stronger in both mind and body; by 1907 Dr Sharp had operated on 176 patients who admitted to having masturbated and claimed that practically all did better at school, slept better, felt better, and had a better appetite. Dr Sharp, an enthusiast, also did 280 vasectomies on patients suffering from colour blindness and defective vision.

Today we have doctors preparing brainwashing techniques for armed forces, fashionable physicians giving slimming drugs to gullible and weak-willed plump ladies; but perhaps worst of all, we have the psychosurgeons.

9. Commercial Research

During the past two decades a good deal of the money spent on medical research has been spent by the pharmaceutical companies. The value of the work done by commercial laboratories is difficult to assess objectively. For various political reasons, research done by the drug industry tends to be either over valued or under-valued, the variation in emphasis depending upon the political inclinations of the commentator concerned or indeed upon his commercial involvement. Observers within the medical profession have been widely divided in their attitudes towards the work done in this way. For example, Lord Platt in his 1967 address to the Royal College of Physicians said that 'The phenomenal success of medical treatment seems to have depended almost wholly on non-clinical and often nonmedical scientists frequently working in, or in close collaboration with, the pharmaceutical industry.' Other doctors (myself included) have accused the drug industry of spending too much money on advertising and developing profitable but medically unnecessary drugs and not enough on doing really useful research. According to a report from the National Economic Development Office 'Focus on Pharmaceuticals', a good proportion of the new drugs put on the market have no advantage over existing ones, they serve only to confuse patients and doctors.

One fact which cannot be disputed is that there have been no real breakthroughs in pharmaceutical research since the 1950s. In a booklet published in 1975 by the Association of the British Pharmaceutical Industry entitled 'Pharmaceutical Research and Public Ownership', the writer, John Maddox, argues that `the past 15 years have seen the introduction of increasingly more specific drugs for the treatment of heart disease, asthma, steroids for the treatment of metabolic diseases as well as for the regulation of fertility.' It is by no means an impressive list when one considers the effort allegedly employed.

As John Maddox in this ABPI publication admits, 'Research programmes costing several million pounds and consuming the energies of dozens of skilled scientists for several years on end are frequently written off as worthless.' He does not admit – but could not deny – that many of the equally expensive research programmes not written off merely produce variations on existing themes. The production of new antacids, tranquillisers and sleeping tablets is seemingly endless.

Most of the money spent on research is spent on searches for products which the companies believe will have a ready sale among doctors. There are a small number of groups of diseases and symptoms which make up a very large proportion of all the work general practitioners do. (Since it is general practitioners who do most of the prescribing in Britain the drug companies aim their efforts largely at them.)

The drug companies seem to me anxious to bring out products which will satisfy two criteria: first that they will be prescribed to a large number of patients, and second that they will be prescribed for long periods of time. Obviously a magical drug which provided a complete cure in one day would not sell in such quantities. So the industry is particularly interested in such conditions as peptic ulceration, iron deficiency anaemia, eczema and psoriasis, obesity, insomnia, and chronic pain such as the pains of arthritis. These are conditions which often need treating for a long period of time and they are also very common.

In the summer of 1975 doctors in the United Kingdom could choose from 57 different brands and varieties of antacid when faced with a patient suffering from gastritis or peptic ulceration. They could prescribe either medicines or tablets and the different compounds all contained slightly different quantities of antacid. But, by and large, the only differences were the names of the products, the names of the manufacturers and the prices.

There is no quick and logical way for the doctor to know which product to prescribe for his patients. He cannot easily compare prices for though these are available, the manufacturers, using all the tricks of the food trade, give prices for different quantities. For example, how do you compare a price of 22 pence for 30 tablets with a price of 87 pence for 300 millilitres? How, indeed, do you compare 22 pence for 30 tablets and 40 pence for 50 tablets? Doctors would need pocket calculators on their desks to be able to ensure that they always prescribed the 'best buy'. And they have no incentive to care.

The companies making those 57 different antacids all promote their products fiercely, they all claim that their version is the best one, and to make matters even more complicated, there is no permanency in the products available. As one product falls out of favour or fails to attract new prescribers, so a new one will be launched by a company anxious to keep its part of the valuable antacid market. The production of these new varieties involves a research project but it is hardly research likely to add usefully to the doctors' armoury of drugs. It will, on the contrary, merely add to their confusion.

The duplication of products continues in all profitable fields. In the summer of 1975 there were 75 different types of iron which could be prescribed by the doctor treating the patient with iron deficiency. These different types of iron were available in different forms, it is true – some as tablets, some as capsules and some for injection. But they were all designed to do exactly the same job. Similarly, there were 15 different types of spermicidal contraceptive waiting to be prescribed, 33 different types of oral contraceptive, 23 different preparations for patients with acne, 103 preparations for patients needing a topical steroid (these drugs are used for patients with long-lasting conditions such as eczema and psoriasis which need semi-continuous therapy and are therefore potentially very profitable), 17 drugs for patients trying to lose weight, 33 drugs for patients unable to sleep, 34 for patients complaining of nausea and sickness and 100 for patients with pain.

In most of these areas one or two branded products would have been quite enough. The amount of research involved in producing all these different products must have been enormous. The companies will have had to try out a new formulation which they can claim will do something no other formulation does; they will then have had to make sure that the combination is not obviously lethal, and that it does indeed sometimes do the job it is supposed to do. When drug companies talk with pride about the amount of money they are spending on research, this is what they are talking about.

The number of products of real value produced in recent years is insignificant compared to the number of products marketed. In fact, it is difficult to think of products introduced in the last two decades which would be missed. Any experienced doctor asked to pick the eight drugs he would choose to take with him on a desert island would choose drugs which have been around for many decades, not because these are the drugs which have been well tried but simply because these are the drugs which work best. Apart from the discovery of sulphonamide, penicillin, steroids, chlorpromazine and insulin in the first half of this century, there have been relatively few discoveries of real note. The drug companies produce hundreds of different products for heart conditions these days but still by far the most important and widely prescribed is digitalis, which has been in use for two centuries. The two most important pain-relieving drugs are aspirin for mild pain, and morphine for more severe pain. These two drugs have been in existence in different forms for centuries although the aspirin tablet as we know it now was not marketed until the end of the nineteenth century. The drug industry has spent much money on producing variations on these two themes but the improvements and additions could hardly be described as revolutionary. Effective antibiotics, analgesics, sedatives and hypnotics were available in the early 1950s. The drug companies are, however, naturally unwilling to admit that the pharmacological revolution is over and that instead of more spectacular discoveries there will merely be the proliferation of products offering marginal advantages to small numbers of patients.

Much drug company money is being spent on research for new drugs which will help relieve anxiety and depression. The drugs so far discovered have been of equivocal value. Nothing has made the same impact as chlorpromazine in the 1950s. There are many different new drugs which have little more value than placebos. They are manufactured and prescribed, however, because this is a fashionable area and one in which there is a great potential for money making. The drug companies which produced the first effective drugs for use against infectious diseases started a gold rush which is still in full flow. Any company that can produce a drug which has a real effect on one or other of the common mental conditions knows that it will make a fortune. Doctors and the industry are both happy to ignore the ethical problems which the discovery of such a drug would produce.

Vast amounts of money have also been spent on the search for a drug with which to attack cancer. So far the drugs which have been produced have only been used on small numbers of patients, though there have been occasional claims that an effective anti-cancer drug is likely to become available. What will probably happen in the next few years will be the promotion of anti-cancer drugs to general practitioners. There is much evidence to show that drug companies have no compunction whatsoever about promoting drugs which may be dangerous, if they think they can make money. There is undoubting big market for these drugs and it will be easy to argue that the drugs will have to be prescribed for long periods of time. Anti-cancer drugs, therefore, fit well into the pattern of drugs suitable for heavy promotion to general practitioners.

In their attempts to produce revolutionary compounds which will match the impact made by the first antibiotics and the first steroids, the drug companies have developed and sold a number of very dangerous substances which they have encouraged doctors to prescribe widely on the basis of limited trials.

The case history of the drug called Eraldin illustrates quite well the problems that have resulted from enthusiastic promotion campaigns. Eraldin is the trade name for a substance called practolol which was originally said to be a potentially important weapon in the war against heart disease. It was recommended for use in patients with angina and in patients with an irregular heart-beat. It was advertised to general practitioners who see thousands of such patients every day and prescribed in vast quantities. It is made by Imperial Chemical Industries.

The dangers of Eraldin first became apparent in 1970/71 when according to a volume entitled *Register of Adverse Reactions*, published by the Committee on Safety of Medicines, a number of side effects were reported. It was not until 1974, however, that the Committee issued any warning to doctors.

Despite the evidence of its dangers the manufacturers, Imperial Chemical Industries, claimed in the 1975 edition of the *Data Sheet Compendium* (a book published by the ABPI which contains prescribing information on drugs available to doctors in Britain) that side effects are 'uncommon' with Eraldin at the recommended dosage. After a number of reports from unhappy prescribers, however, ICI eventually announced in July 1975 that from October 1975 the drug would only be available to hospitals. Even in September 1975 a cardiologist, at a meeting at the Warwickshire Postgraduate Education Centre attended by physicians and general practitioners from all over the country, referred to a recently completed and shortly to be published trial of practolol which had shown how useful it was. He failed to mention, however, that it had also been shown that practolol caused severe damage to eyes, cars, kidneys, skin and intestines. It seems quite likely that though this drug has, to all intents and purposes, been banned, it will still be prescribed occasionally by some physicians. This drug was a member of a group with great earning potential and many of ICI's competitors are still promoting their own variations on this particular theme.

Some of the drugs promoted are pharmacologically identical but were given different brand names because of licensing arrangements between different companies. For example, the drug sotalol was marketed as 'Sotacor' by Bristol Laboratories and as 'Beta-Cardone' by Duncan, Flockhart, and the substance metoprolol was marketed as 'Betaloc' by Astra, and as 'Lopressor' by Geigy. All these products came onto the market just as 'Eraldin' was being withdrawn and were described by their manufacturers and distributors as being safe alternatives.

Lack of research evidence relating specifically to these drugs made it possible for the companies to make these claims but in September 1975 the Committee on Safety of Medicines published the first of a series of leaflets entitled 'Current Problems' which included a note on such drugs and others in the same group. The note pointed out that these drugs may cause the same problems as Eraldin. At about the same time researchers from the University of California, writing in the *New England Journal of Medicine* reported that two patients out of twenty died when they were taken off one of the drugs in this particular group. Other writers in the same *Journal* pointed out that it is very possible that the problems produced by Eraldin will be produced in due course by all the alternatives.

There is plenty of evidence to show that drug companies are much more concerned with doing research that will help to sell products than in doing research to ensure that products are safe and effective. I described the evidence in greater detail in my book *The Medicine Men* (published in 1975).

Hospital and general practice trials are often done by doctors working for the company which has made the drug under trial. Even if the doctors concerned are contractually employed outside the company there is a very good chance that they will be paid a fee for their work. In America hospitals charge drug companies for each case record supplied. The charge of about 2,000 dollars for each record can mount up to a quarter of a million dollars for enough records to make a complete trial. In European hospitals outside Britain the charges are rather lower than this – and in Britain they are much lower, with the doctors accepting a free dinner, a piece of equipment or a ticket to a conference abroad as a reward. The size of the reward is unimportant: the fact is that when inducements are offered to doctors, the doctors become, effectively, employees of the companies concerned and their reports must inevitably be considered bearing that fact in mind.

Another worrying aspect of the testing of drug company products is the fact that patients are rarely told that they are taking part in a trial when they are given drugs by their general practitioner or hospital consultant. They may be told that the doctor has something new for them to try and the doctor himself may be under the impression that he is handing out a well-tried product which merely needs proving in clinical practice. In fact he may well be giving a potentially lethal drug to patients who will be out of his sight for a week at a time.

There is another result of the drug companies' need to publicise their products and ensure that the information they think relevant reaches the maximum number of doctors. As a writer in *General Practitioner*, one of the free circulation medical magazines, put it, 'For the drug companies the need to publish information overrides considerations like the circulation of the journal or its editorial standards.' The reason for this is that the drug companies know that few prescribers actually read any of the articles in the medical journals. What the drug companies want are references to quote on their attractive give-away literature and for their representatives to quote when visiting general practitioners.

Again in the words of *General Practitioner*, 'The medical reference is the most trusty weapon in the drug company representative's armoury. Quoting chapter and verse on a published clinical trial gives an air of respectability to his claims, which are then harder for the doctor to question...'

This would be all very well if the drug companies only published in journals such as *British Medical Journal*, *The Lancet* and so on. The drug companies do not, however, publish their findings only in these established journals. They also publish in journals which actually charge the companies a fee – said to be about £500 for an article of average length.

The *Journal of International Medical Research*, for example, was in September 1975 charging £85 per printed page for scientific papers published in it. According to the publishers, In addition to publishing medical and scientific papers the *Journal of International Medical Research* also undertakes the recording, transcription and publication of symposia, under its imprint; with, where necessary, the translation of the proceedings into languages other than English.

For example Volume 3 Supplement 3 of the *Journal* includes the proceedings of an International Vivalan Symposium held at the Cunard International Hotel, London. This symposium was attended by 28 foreign employees of Imperial Chemical Industries Ltd, the manufacturers of Vivalan (an antidepressant drug), 78 doctors from Argentina, Australia, Belgium, Brazil, Denmark, Eire, Finland, France, Germany, Holland, Italy, Japan, Mexico, Norway, Poland, Portugal, Sweden, Switzerland and Yugoslavia, and 110 doctors from different parts of the United Kingdom. There are 125 pages in the *Journal* Supplement referring to Vivalan and these pages include papers given by Dr Eric Murphy, the Editor in Chief of the *Journal*, and Dr Bayliss of the Clinical Research Department of Imperial Chemical Industries.

When I wrote to IC for prescribing information about Vivalan, I was sent a typically colourful and well-produced brochure describing in the usual glowing terms the work done, proving how effective and unique Vivalan is. The vivid prose was based largely on twelve references listed in the back of the brochure in proper scientific fashion. The majority of these references dealt with information made available at the Vivalan Symposium and published in the *Journal of International Medical Research*. Few GPs see the Journal and even fewer know that companies buy space in it to publish their papers. But they do see – and accept as genuine – the references to the Journal which appear in advertising literature.

Researchers are so delighted to have their work published that they will happily agree to let drug companies pay for the work to appear in journals of lesser standing. And even members of the medical profession appear to give their approval to the whole business by allowing their names to be used as members of the editorial boards of these journals. *The Journal of International Medical Research*, for example, includes on its United Kingdom editorial board Professor J.P. Payne, Professor W. Linford Rees and Professor Andrew Semple.

The research into new drugs is also beset with many ethical problems. Difficulties may arise, for example, if a new drug is discovered which, though excellent in itself, has no marketing advantage over competitors' products. And it is not unknown for a company to develop a product which has advantages over existing drugs but to refrain from marketing it because they already have a market leader and see no point in competing with themselves.

There is no doubt that the commercial drug companies have in the last three-quarters of a century put onto the market a number of extremely important drugs. Much of the most important medical research done this century has been financed by drug companies. However, the evidence now suggests convincingly that the drug companies are unlikely to continue producing useful drugs at a similar rate in the future. Most of the drugs being put onto the market today are merely variations on existing themes and the drug companies are doing themselves irreparable harm in their attempts to promote these products. There is no medical justification for the continued expenditure of vast amounts of money on traditional research by the drug companies. In a later chapter I shall explain what I think the drug companies should be researching.

10. Ethical Problems Today

As scientists progress and increase our knowledge and technical skills so they create more and more ethical problems. Questions are raised about just how far doctors should go to prolong life and the dangers their creations often produce. However, it is in the collection of information that medical researchers most commonly offend. After all, a researcher cannot be held entirely responsible for all the effects of his work but he must be held responsible for the way he does his research.

The doctor who takes on the responsibility for the health of a human being has a duty to ensure that no unnecessary diagnostic tests are performed and no treatments initiated which may lower the patient's chances of survival and cure. As the Frenchman, Claud Bernard, put it, 'It is our duty and our right to perform an experiment on man whenever it can save his life, cure him, or gain him some personal benefit. The principle of medical and surgical morality, therefore, consists in never performing on man an experiment which might be harmful to him to any extent, even though the result might be highly advantageous to science, that is, to the health of others.' It is equally true, of course, to say that the doctor has a responsibility to learn from the treatment of each patient, to accumulate knowledge and to apply what he learns to the treatment of others.

Before discussing unnecessary experiments on patients, it is necessary to define an 'experiment'. According to Henry K. Beecher, an experiment may be defined as weighing a baby unnecessarily, taking a few drops of blood too much from a patient so that unnecessary tests can be done, and giving any drug to any patient. Certainly today diagnostic and therapeutic techniques are so complex and technical that almost every case is an experiment. Certainly giving a drug is always an experiment; no one can be sure about the result.

Experiments can be done on unknowing patients who are in hospital for treatment, on healthy volunteers who agree to be used in an experiment for some reason although they do not require treatment, and on sick patients who have agreed to take part in an experimental study. Researchers may also experiment on themselves and many often do. The experiments which most often prove worrying and which are most likely to concern the average man are those which concern the patient in hospital or in a doctor's surgery. These experiments can be divided into two important groups: those in which something unnecessary is done and those in which something necessary is not done.

According to Beecher 'Of 100 consecutive human studies published in 1964 in an excellent journal, 12 seemed to be unethical.' The British clinician Pappworth has collected over 500 papers based upon unethical experimentation. Many of these dubious experiments are performed by young doctors anxious to prove themselves, publish research papers and acquire an academic background which will help them advance in their profession. There has been for a long time a great deal of emphasis on the importance of research as a prelude to a position of responsibility within a hospital, and there is in addition a great deal of money available for such work. The combination of these factors means that much research of doubtful validity is done by researchers who lack the necessary sense of responsibility. Undoubtedly many are also thoughtless and careless, thinking more about themselves than their patients. Part of the responsibility for this sad state of affairs must certainly lie with those who train doctors for there is good evidence to show that many doctors have never been properly made aware of the dangers of unethical trials, and never fully acquainted with their responsibilities as researchers.

In one hospital survey 26 normal babies less than 48 hours old were subjected to X-rays while their bladders were filled. The examination carried no possible advantage for the babies but a definite risk to their health. In another American study, live cancer cells were injected into 22 human subjects as part of a study of immunity to cancer. The patients concerned were not told what was happening. In an investigation into the effects of the removal of the thymus gland, 18 children who were about to have surgery for congenital heart disease were selected and 11 were chosen to have their thymus gland removed. There was no advantage to the children in this additional surgery and there could well have been dangerous disadvantages. These and many other trials which are equally horrifying are quoted in an article by Henry K. Beecher, Dorr

Professor of Research in Anaesthesia at Harvard Medical School, entitled 'Ethics and Clinical Research' which was published in the *New England Journal of Medicine* on 16 June 1966. References are not given in the article since Beecher claims that he has no intention of pointing to individuals, but the editors of the *New England Journal* were satisfied by Beecher's unpublished list of references.

In many hospitals pregnant women undergo routine investigations which enable their gynaecologists to assess new methods of anaesthesia. It is true that such a new method, if it works, may benefit many women but what about the women having babies who are subjected to tests with a method which does not work or which turns out to have dangerous side effects as some tests have done? Numerous papers have been published which confirm that new methods of anaesthesia may prove dangerous but the following papers provide a good selection: 'Foetal heart rate patterns following epidural anaesthesia and oxytocin infusion during labour' by Barry S. Schifrin of the Beth Israel Hospital, Harvard Medical School, who published his paper in the *Journal of Obstetrics and Gynaecology of the British Commonwealth* in April 1972; 'The effects of epidural analgesia upon foetal and neonatal status' by Wingate, Wingate, Iffy, Freundlich and Gottsegen of Thomas Jefferson University and Philadelphia Hospital, Philadelphia, Pennsylvania, published in the *American Journal of Obstetrics and Gynecology* on 15 August 1974; 'Epidural analgesia for obstetrics' by McDonald, Bjorkman and Reed of Los Angeles, California, published in the *American Journal of Obstetrics and Gynecology* on 15 December 1974; 'The Foetal influence of continuous lumbar epidural analgesia in labour' by Thiery, De Clercq, Rolly, Derom, Vroman and Diesbecq, published in *Acta Anaesthesiologica Belgica* in January 1974. All these papers seem to suggest that doctors should be cautious about offering new techniques to women in labour. Nevertheless, these new techniques are offered frequently.

In a paper entitled *Pelvic Arteriography in Obstetrics* published in the *American Journal of Obstetrics and Gynecology* in January 1961, Solish, Masterson and Hellman from Brooklyn, New York, describe a number of experiments performed on pregnant women. In several cases the women concerned went into labour early.

Robert F. Heimburger MD, C. Courtney Whitlock MD and John E. Kalsbeck MD of the Indiana University Medical 'Centre,

Indianapolis, used stereotaxic amygdalotomy (a type of brain surgery) to treat 25 patients between the ages of 7 and 61. These patients were described as having episodic or constant hostile, aggressive and destructive behaviour; two 15-year-old girls were specifically described as 'aggressive'. The results of this work were published in the *Journal of the American Medical Association* in November 1966.

At Northwick Park Hospital in England, according to an adulatory article in a British medical magazine, experiments are continuing into cerebral blood flow. According to one journalist, '... the patient breathes in radioactive xenon in oxygen for ten minutes ... the radioactive gas which he has been inhaling is taken up by the blood stream and passes into the brain. The changes in the radioactivity within the cerebral blood vessels are picked up by the sensors alongside the patient's head.' The writer admitted that some of the patients 'must be a little overawed, if not sometimes frightened, by the amount of investigative work which is done on them by the complex and advanced equipment with which they are confined.'

During a recent Medical Research Council trial on the best ways to treat patients with hypertension, patients were, according to Dr C.T. Dollery of the Royal Postgraduate Medical School, London, tested for 'compliance'. In other words an experiment was conducted to find out just how many patients were taking the pills they were prescribed. The experiment involved the taking of blood from patients. This is not a particularly painful or dangerous procedure but it is one which worries many patients and for doctors to assume that its use is justified simply because an experiment is being conducted is disturbing. Those patients involved in the MRC trial stood to gain nothing at all from the experiment, but their permission was not obtained.

Doctors in many centres have recently been performing operations on patients wishing to lose weight. Unable to help patients with dietary advice, with drugs or by wiring their jaws together, surgeons have now developed an operation which involves cutting out a large amount of intestine to create an artificial malabsorption syndrome. The operation involves joining up the top end of the gut directly to the bottom end. The theory is that any food eaten will simply hurtle through and no stop long enough to be digested and absorbed. Apart from the facts that the operation (a dangerous one to perform) does not always work, that when it does, the weight loss usually stops after a year or eighteen months and that all the evidence suggests that patients only lose weight because, with so little room in their intestines, they have a 'full' feeling sooner, there are a number of real dangers. Dr T.R.E. Pilkington of St George's Hospital, London, has reported three deaths due to the operation and Mr Baddeley at the General Hospital, Birmingham, has reported severe trouble, with some patients suffering from liver damage and metabolic problems. It seems a very heavy price to pay and, once again, this must stand as another example of research work creating clinical problems.

In a book entitled *Curiosa*, William St Clair Symmers describes how a young mother, admitted to a medical ward for the investigation of symptoms suggestive of a gastric ulcer, was subjected to cardiac catheterisation, a hazardous procedure. No specific permission was obtained and there was no clinical reason at all to perform the experiment. Unfortunately for the patient the catheter used for the experiment got stuck inside her and had to be removed by a thoracic surgeon.

In May 1975 surgeons at Harefield Hospital, Uxbridge, Middlesex, kept a 13-month-old boy alive for 16 hours by connecting him to the heart, lungs and kidneys of a baboon. The operation was carried out after the child's heart and lungs had failed following an operation for a congenital heart defect. The animal eventually died, killed by toxic materials in the boy's blood. The surgeon did not regard the operation as a failure for, as he pointed out, he had prolonged a life. As the medical consultant to the *Daily Telegraph* commented, 'There is apparently no limit today to the extent to which surgeons will go in an attempt to maintain life – no matter how remote may be the chances of that life being of any value to the individual concerned.'

Errors of omission can sometimes be just as serious as errors of commission. For example, there have been many trials involving drugs in which patients have *not* been given drugs of first choice so that new theories can be tried out. These trials can, of course, be just as unethical as trials in which new and dangerous procedures are tested, for the patient who does not receive a life-saving treatment and dies has been poorly treated by his attendants.

In 1932, for example, a number of negroes in Alabama with syphilis were given no treatment at all so that the course of untreated syphilis could be followed all the way to insanity, heart disease, paralysis and premature death. Even when penicillin was introduced and found to cure syphilis, these negroes were deprived of it so that the experiment was not spoiled.

The alternative to using real patients when performing experiments is sometimes to use volunteers. As long as an experiment does not call for the use of patients with specific lesions or symptoms, then healthy volunteers can occasionally be of service. Many researchers believe strongly in the use of volunteers and recruit wherever they can. Traditionally volunteers can usually be found in prisons. In ancient Persia condemned criminals would sometimes be handed over to doctors for use in medical experiments. In 1722 inmates of Newgate Prison volunteered to be inoculated with smallpox as an alternative to hanging. They lived and were freed. Similar incentives are common today. Pardons and reprieves, offered or implied, can sometimes be obtained and prisoners are popular material for researchers because there are large numbers of people available in one place in an environment which can be accurately controlled. One pair of researchers alone, using 224 prisoners, have published over 80 scientific articles. Prisoners can be followed for months or even years, they can be given strict diets, allowed fixed amounts of exercise and so on.

Volunteers volunteer for many reasons. Prisoners may volunteer because they see a shorter sentence. Other subjects volunteer for altruistic reasons or simply for money. Some may not really know what they are doing. Experiments on lunatics were first performed (officially) in 1905 when William Fletcher took patients in an asylum at Kuala Lumpur into the asylum dining-room and divided them into two groups. Half were given uncured rice and half had cured rice. Forty-three of the 120 people in the second group developed beriberi and 18 of these died.

According to a *Daily Telegraph* report in August 1975, a 42-year-old man, a patient at the New York Psychiatric Institute, was in 1953 given drugs by the American Army as part of a 29 day project when the Institute had given the Army a contract to conduct experiments on its inmates to 'determine the clinical effects of psycho-chemical agents on the psychiatric behaviour of human subjects'. The man died and his death was officially reported as being due to heart failure.

Soldiers, sailors and airmen are often used as guinea pigs. They can be easily controlled, easily kept in one place and easily subjected to the strict discipline necessary for a research project. It is usually suggested in ethical codes that no serving members of armed forces should ever be involved in experiments, since professional warriors have little chance of refusing a request for volunteers. However, it does seem that forces personnel are used in experimental work.

In an article entitled 'It's a research worker's dream' which appeared in the medical magazine *Doctor* in Britain, in March 1975 a writer, describing the Institute of Naval Medicine at Alverstoke in Hampshire, wrote that 'Soon to be published is the result of the last experimental series to ascertain the acceptable safety level for continuous exposure of man to carbon dioxide.' The writer also pointed out that studies are currently under way to investigate ways of protecting patients against radiation. One presumes that the subjects of these experiments are volunteers but cannot help wondering how much choice service personnel have when volunteering and how much they understand exactly what is going on.

Attempts to obtain permission from volunteers are not always wholehearted and some volunteers may not thoroughly understand what they are doing. Few people will risk their lives for science and so the most dangerous experiments must be performed without explaining fully the risks or by taking advantage of the volunteers' mental state.

One study done by Lasagna and von Felsinger showed that those who volunteer for experiment may not be normal. Of 56 male college student volunteers between the ages of 21 and 28, 25 had psychological problems and had volunteered for 'kicks' or because of self-destructive urges. Other studies have also shown that 50 per cent of volunteers have psychological problems. The actual request for consent may so upset the potential volunteer that he or she is not sure what he or she is doing. And of course, since doctors still have a great deal of public trust, many people will accept reassurances happily and agree to take part in experiments simply because they do not believe that any doctor could subject a human being to appreciable risk.

Even unsuspecting and perfectly healthy people may occasionally find themselves victims of ruthless scientists looking for guinea pigs. This sounds over-dramatic, but consider biochemist Dr Frank Olsen who leapt from a tenth-floor hotel window in America after CIA scientists had given him LSD without his knowledge. Over 500 unwitting subjects are now known to have been involved in US Army experiments during the last two decades.

Much medical research is now done in developing countries and those with suspicious minds say that the reason is that rules there are not so strict about the performing of trials on patients or healthy volunteers.

Those who have such faith in human nature that they believe that only the dramatically sick could deliberately subject fellow human beings to real risk should read the reports of Stanley Migram who published, in a book entitled `Obedience to Authority', details of extraordinary experiments he conducted while he was Assistant Professor of Psychology at Yale University. He invited a number of ordinary men and women from Newhaven to help in research into punishment and learning and offered a payment of 4 dollars plus travelling expenses. The volunteers came to the laboratory and were told that the experiments were a study into memory and learning. Each volunteer was told that one person would act as 'teacher' and the other as 'pupil'. The 'pupil' was put into a chair and an electrode fastened to each wrist. He was given a list of word pairs to learn and told that he would get shocks of increasing intensity if he made errors. The 'pupil' was in fact an actor and the electrodes were fake. The 'teacher' was the only real subject in the experiment. The 'pupil' pretended to be in pain when the shocks were given and when the teachers hesitated to give further shocks the person in charge of the experiment instructed them to get on with things. 'The main question', according to Migram, was `how far the participant would comply with the experimenter's instructions before refusing to carry out the actions required...'.

The 'teachers' were all ordinary people and almost two-thirds kept giving shocks obediently, disregarding the screams of pain from the 'pupil'. If people with no real interest in an experiment can get so carried away, how much more can those with a real career involvement.

I can illustrate vividly the dilemma faced by the clinician who does research. I recently talked to a physician interested in research into liver damage caused by paracetamol poisoning. He confessed that to his own horror he had found himself welcoming the admission to hospital of a patient who had taken an overdose of paracetamol and moaning because the patient had been sick and thereby more or less ensured that his liver would remain undamaged: a painful illustration of the conflict between the aims of the clinician and the ambitions of the researchers.

As Hugo Glaser reports in *The Drama of Medicine* many medical researchers, either unable or unwilling to find volunteers or suitable patients for their experiments, have used themselves as experimental subjects. In 1830, for example, to show the French Academy and to convince them of the accuracy of his claim that charcoal would absorb alkalis, a scientist called Tonery took a potentially lethal dose of strychnine and charcoal.

Some of the most daring research has been done on infectious diseases. A German called Pettenkofer, trying to understand just how cholera attacked the human body, swallowed millions of cholera germs in 1892. Because he suspected that the acid juices of the stomach would kill off the bacilli he even swallowed an alkali mixture to make sure that the bacilli stood a fair chance. He did not learn anything but his bravery must be admired. About a century earlier a British doctor, Dr A. White, deliberately infected himself with bubonic plague. He took some of the discharge from a patient's suppurating gland and rubbed it into his own thigh. The next day he made a cut in his forearm and put some of the suppurating matter into the wound. Eight days later White died. He had proved his point about the infective nature of bubonic plague.

Leprosy is a disease which frightens many people but in the mid-nineteenth century a Norwegian doctor, Daniel Danielssen, made a number of experiments on himself, in an attempt to discover just how infectious leprosy is and whether people are justified in shunning lepers. In fact leprosy is not very infectious, but before he had satisfied himself of this, Danielssen had injected himself with matter from a leprous nodule and even cut off a piece of a patient's nodule and implanted it under his own skin. That would be a brave action for a man who knew that leprosy was not highly infectious;

for someone who did not know for certain, it was an extraordinary thing to do.

In 1767 John Hunter, one of the most famous surgeons of all time, took some of the discharge from a man with venereal disease and put it into his own urinary tract. In 1851 a young German doctor put matter from a patient with secondary syphilis into a superficial wound on his arm. Both these doctors suffered a great deal.

There have, according to Hugo Glaser, been many brave experiments performed by researchers on themselves during the last few decades. In 1928 a Dr Werner Forssmann made a cut in a vein at his elbow and introduced through the cut a long catheter which he pushed in the direction of his heart. He introduced 26 inches of tube and got it as far as the right side of his heart. With the aid of this tube he managed to show that the pressure inside the heart could be measured. Much modern heart surgery is based on these simple experiments.

In May 1933 a Swiss doctor, Dr Jacques Pontot, let himself be bitten by three adders. He had developed a serum against snake bite which he wanted to demonstrate. In January 1950 a Polish woman doctor Clara Fonti, working in Italy, decided on an experiment which she thought might help to prove that cancer is caused by a virus. She opened her blouse and rubbed one of her breasts against the breast of another woman with a fungating cancer which had broken through the skin. Though there was no transmission of the cancer, Dr Fonti developed serious blood poisoning.

In 1958 Dr Barrera Oro, working in Buenos Aires, injected himself with a culture produced from a virus of a newly discovered disease. Before doing this he wrote a letter to the Dean of the university, ruling that no one should interfere or try to stop the disease developing. It did develop, was treated and the young doctor survived, though it was a close thing for a while. Dr Oro and his colleagues obtained vital information from this experiment.

There have been many attempts to formulate powerful ethical codes to help researchers decide what action they should or should not take under a given set of circumstances. But, as Dr Irvine H. Page of Cleveland wrote in the *Journal of the American Medical Association* in April 1975, 'The current literature on human experimentation is so filled with claims, counter claims and confusion I would seriously doubt that most physicians or researchers are able either to understand the problems or to follow the supposedly clarifying guidelines.' The plain fact is that whatever ethical codes are formulated and whatever is said to be 'morally responsible' and 'ethical', there will always be researchers who prefer to follow their own inclinations and ignore the pleadings of those they consider to be opposed to progress. In a study of medical researchers it was found that only 6 per cent of them gave 'ethical concern for research subjects' as one of three essential factors they would look for when choosing a research associate. Large numbers of researchers seemed happy to conduct almost any research without the subject's permission, so long as they thought there was a chance that something of use would come out of the research.

In view of this, it seems that in order to control researchers we need to adopt controls they will understand. One of the most powerful of these would surely be a proper control over publication. In 1955 the Public Health Council of the Netherlands stated that 'Publication of articles describing human experiments that are contrary to medical ethics is strongly criticised; and it is recommended that medical journals refuse to publish articles based on unethical experiments.'

Unfortunately, the editors of most international journals still believe that if unethical research has been done it is better to publish the research and so at least justify the risks to which subjects have been exposed. Editors will also argue that if they do not publish, someone else will. It is interesting to note that the US Supreme Court recently stated that 'evidence unconstitutionally obtained cannot be used in any judicial decision, no matter how important the evidence is to the ends of justice'.

I believe that in order to improve the ethics of our researchers, a number of steps must be taken. Every experiment planned should be explained to the subjects concerned by an independent clinician, that is, one not concerned with the experiment. Links between industry and researchers are dangerous and should be severed completely. I would like to see all full-time researchers removed from the medical register and only registered practitioners allowed to conduct trials involving human beings. In this way patients could be assured that only practising clinicians, subject to the usual professional codes, could be involved in clinical research.

Medical ethics should receive more attention in medical schools and students should be taught to be suspicious of any experiment and to ask, first and foremost, So what? and then, Will this experiment help my patient? No harmful experiment which does not contribute to the individual patient's welfare can be justified. At the present time 'medical ethics' are ignored in most medical schools.

Medical researchers create and get involved in many other areas where there are real ethical problems. Much research, for example, involves the use of medical records originally kept by doctors to help them treat particular patients. When a patient visits a doctor he believes that what he tells the doctor will remain a secret. He knows that the doctor's colleagues and perhaps the doctor's secretary may have to be told some of his secrets, but by and large he trusts the doctor's discretion and is therefore happy to answer just about any questions the doctor wishes to ask. He does not expect that the information he gives will be used for any purpose other than the treatment of his own illness.

However, some of the most important medical discoveries of recent years have been made by the study of medical records. Researchers have studied the incidence of specific diseases in specific populations and then searched for common factors. By studying medical records, for example, it was possible to show that cigarette smokers have a higher than average incidence of lung cancer.

Much of the information about the chemical and industrial causes of cancer was taken from medical records kept by general practitioners and by hospital doctors. By studying work records it was possible to prove that workers involved in the production of some rubber articles were particularly liable to develop cancer of the bladder. As a result it was possible to help protect some of the other workers who might have been exposed to risk.

The Medical Research Council, which has arranged some of the work using medical records, has stated that 'Medical information obtained about identified individual patients should continue to be made available without their explicit consent for the purposes of medical research.' And so the present situation is that your medical records, which you had previously thought to be inviolable, can now be examined by researchers without your permission being given. Very few general practitioners or consultants would refuse to cooperate with researchers asking for help. The important point is that the patients concerned can be identified – they are not simply medical statistics.

One unfortunate point is that often the researchers involved in epidemiological studies are not medically qualified. Very few are in medical practice. Many are social workers who do not have a strict ethical code to obey. Once information has been made available to social workers, there is no guarantee at all that it will be treated carefully. There is powerful evidence to show that social workers do not even have a carefully developed sense of what is meant by 'confidential'. A social worker reported in April 1975 that 'Researchers posing as social workers were able to get full information about clients from probation officers and social workers over the phone'.

Fortunately I am pleased to say that worry about this problem of confidentiality seems to be spreading. Mrs Shirley Williams pointed out in a recent House of Commons debate that 'It needs only a moment's imagination to realise if one could link up medical records with employment records in such a way as to reveal, for instance, past treatment for psychiatric illness or venereal diseases, how widely we are extending the power over individuals in a way that frankly I find extremely disturbing.'

Speaking at a meeting of the British Association for the Advancement of Science in September 1975, Dr Dolton, regional specialist in community medicine with the Mersey Regional Health Authority talked of his worries about the increasing amount of data collected from patients by doctors which is eventually stored in computers and in data banks of other kinds and which can be used for medical research or simply as a check on the patient himself. Dr Dolton recalled as examples the ethical problems created by a child-minder with gonorrhoea, a schoolteacher with a driving licence who had epilepsy, a publican with tuberculosis and a homosexual who wanted to adopt a child. All these people had originally offered themselves to a doctor for treatment. Their medical records had been stored for their benefit and for the benefit of future medical attendants and researchers.

I am afraid that, as a general practitioner, I have now decided that not only will I refuse to provide social workers, personnel officers, lawyers and policemen with any information about my patients unless the patient expressly asks me to provide it, but that I will also refuse to provide information to anyone conducting a research programme, and refuse to make my records available to anyone not providing the patient concerned with medical aid of some essential sort. I receive fairly regular requests for information from doctors organising research but all such requests go straight into my waste-paper basket. My concern as a general practitioner must be with my patients now, not with the next generation of patients.

An ethical problem which arouses as much public interest as any other is the use of animals for research purposes. Those who support the use of animals argue that, without studies on animals, most of the advances in the prevention, diagnosis and treatment of disease would never have been made. It would, they say, have been impossible to conduct the same trials on human beings.

Those who oppose the use of animals in research, on a logical rather than an emotional basis, do so purely on the grounds that too many animals are used and that much unnecessary research is done. The use of animals is so widespread now that there is even a danger that some species will be wiped out. About a quarter of a million primates are used every year in medical research, and though some are specially bred, many are captured from the wild. One and a half million rhesus monkeys were used during the years 1954/60 in the United States alone. According to an article in the *British Veterinary Journal* in October 1972 by E.G. Hartley of the National Institute for Medical Research in London, 'In certain areas of India in which the rhesus population was high some years ago few are now to be found.' Hartley also wrote that No one can deny that some effect on the conservation of certain primate species has been caused by the large number of primates captured annually for biochemical research purposes.' According to the Home Office over 5¼ million animal experiments are performed each year in Britain alone. It is estimated that up to 200 million experiments on living animals are performed in the USA each year.

Some of the most thoughtful comments on animal experiments have come from medical researchers themselves. In an interview published in the medical magazine *Interface*, researcher Denis Burkitt described how, when a friend of his at the Medical Research Council received a proposal for a research project, he would write 'So what?' at the end of it.

`Now although I realise and accept the need for animal experimentation,' said Burkitt, 'I think that to inflict a lot of suffering on animals purely to satisfy curiosity, when there are going to be no fairly obvious predictable results – no answer to the question So What? – then I think this can get you into a line which could be immoral and perhaps unjustified.'

Researcher Richard D. Ryder, in *Victims of Science* pointed out that the horror drug thalidomide was tested rigorously on animals, and that, even after it had proved to have such disastrous effects in humans, it was exceedingly difficult to reproduce the effects in animals in the laboratory. His point is that the animal tests done on thalidomide did not protect us from the drug. He also makes the point that insulin produces deformities in chickens, rabbits and mice and that cortisone produces deformities in mice.

In past years most of the opposition to animal research has been squashed easily by researchers who have complained righteously that the complaints are made by people who love animals more than human beings. A Cambridge psychologist who removed a monkey's visual cortex and kept the blinded monkey for six years so that he could study her, replied to comments accusing him of cruelty by pointing out that some people just wanted to stop research. Researchers, it seems, can follow their own rules as long as they are researching.

Certainly very little of the suffering inflicted on animals in the name of medical science has had much to do with actual medical practice. As Ryder showed, many tests are done for purely commercial purposes and firms making cosmetics often have large laboratories where animals are poisoned systematically with cosmetics in order to complete toxicological studies. Researchers have deprived animals of food and water, subjected some to pain and attempted to terrify others. Many of the experiments performed unnecessarily are done by students who could easily learn from filmed experiments or from well-illustrated text books. While at medical school I was expected to perform vivisection experiments which could only have been condoned by cruel and unthinking people. (For the record, I refused.)

The present-day ethical problems which I have so far discussed are ones which have been around for many years. Opposition to research involving the use of animals is no new phenomenon, neither is opposition to the use of human beings in potentially dangerous research programmes. There are, however, a number of ethical problems facing doctors today which were unknown a generation ago. One of the most important topical problems which has resulted from the efforts of medical researchers is the difficulty of knowing when a patient has died and when to let a patient die. There are machines capable of taking over the functions of the heart and lungs and though the brain may be irreversibly damaged, blood may continue to flow round the body. The case of General Franco who eventually died late in 1975 after having been kept alive for several weeks after most ordinary citizens would have been pronounced dead illustrates the capability of modern machinery.

Hospital doctors are often placed in a difficult situation. If they let a patient die they could, in theory, be accused of murder or manslaughter. Relatives might be tempted to begin lawsuits and so naturally the tendency is to keep every patient alive for as long as possible with the equipment available. Even the 90-year-old patient with no hope for the future will be given the full treatment if he has a heart attack in hospital. Many old people find all this so worrying that they are reluctant to go into hospital at all. Charles Lindbergh was lucky enough to be able to spend his last few days on a beautiful island. Many other old people are not so lucky; they die with tubes emerging from every orifice and without any dignity or peace.

Relatives sometimes find it most distressing to have to stand by and watch while a relative is kept alive in an intensive care unit. Frequently patients with brain damage have been kept alive for months or even ears when there has been no hope of recovery. In autumn 1975 a court in New Jersey was asked by the father of a 21-year-old girl who had been in a coma for five months to allow her to die. The girl had irreparable brain damage but the doctors, worried lest they be charged with manslaughter, would not turn the machine off.

It is also difficult to know when a patient has died. Today electrocardiographs and electroencephalograms have been introduced to provide doctors with mechanical ways of defining death. However, these machines produce as many problems as they solve, for a patient who is dead according to the electroencephalogram may still be alive according to the electrocardiogram. And vice versa. This particular problem is intensified for surgeons working in the transplant field. They have to decide when a donor has actually died and when his organs can be removed and their decisions have to be made within seconds. In the United Kingdom all vital functions must stop before an organ can be removed, but in France brain death is all-important and surgeons will happily and legally remove a patient's kidneys while his heart is still beating. A Euro transplant system was set up to exchange donor organs between countries, but it quickly ground to a halt because organs available in the United Kingdom are considered useless in France and organs from France are considered in Britain to have been illegally obtained.

The time of death is important, because the transplant surgeon has to snatch the organs he will put into the recipient as soon as the donor has died. If the organs are left too long in a decaying body they will become useless. The kidneys for example, are no good when they are cold and no longer perfused with blood. In practice this means that the patient must be kept 'artificially alive' until the kidneys are removed.

There are, of course, dangers that mistakes will be made. There have been terrifying reports of patients waking up as the surgeon had his knife poised ready. Several such patients have recovered and left the hospital as well as the operating table.

The problem of deciding when a patient has died and when his organs may be removed to help another patient can be well illustrated by describing what happened to a university administrator in Wisconsin who suffered a heart attack early in 1975. By the time he reached hospital he had stopped breathing and he was declared clinically dead. His wife authorised the removal of his eyes and kidneys. Just as he was being wheeled into the operating theatre for the removal operation a nurse noticed that his eyelids were fluttering. The patient was returned to the ward and two days later he sat in a chair and ate his breakfast with his wife. There are many similar examples in the medical literature.

Some British surgeons are, however, unhappy about the fact that they are expected to obtain permission before removing organs from a patient. Originally, it was assumed that a patient did not want to have his organs removed unless he carried a card giving the surgeon permission or unless permission could be obtained from a close relative. Today, however, some surgeons insist that they must have the right to remove a patient's organs without his permission, and to assume that. unless he is carrying a card forbidding such removal, permission has been given. The self-service morgue is here.

According to a report in *General Practitioner* on 2 January 1976, 'Kidney transplant surgeons in Britain have started to remove organs from donors before their hearts have stopped beating, but they are reticent about publicising the practice because of the possibility of arousing controversy.' In another medical magazine, *Medical News*, in the same week, Dr Maurice Rosen wrote that 'The time has come for legislation to enact that, on the death of an individual, that person's organs would become the property of the Health Service, in order to benefit those in need of transplant operations.'

What will happen I wonder, when surgeons begin as a matter of routine to transplant lungs, livers, hearts and other organs? There will be a mad scramble for parts of any patient unlucky enough to die in a hospital and undoubtedly many more patients will insist on being left alone at home to die.

11. Ethical Problems Tomorrow

There have been many attempts to guess what life is going to be like in the future. Today only the gambler or guesser would try to imagine what life will be like more than twenty-five years ahead; it is difficult enough to try and guess what life will be like in five years' time. Those who in the past have tried to make similar forecasts have been proved hopelessly unsuccessful some turning out too optimistic and some too pessimistic. In a book entitled *Medicines in the 1990s – a technological forecast*, published by the drug industry's champion, The Office of Health Economics, in 1969, one writer suggested that `...by 1975 diabetes should be completely and reliably controlled by oral agents.' The same publication also contained the forecast that. more effective long-acting preparations which might improve the blood supply to the heart muscle, and medicines designed to prevent anginal attacks while not depressing the heart muscle will both be developed by 1975 and its authors forecast that by 1975 there should be a 'male pill, a contraceptive pill for taking after intercourse, a long-acting pill, and a technique for immunising against pregnancy'. All these forecasts have been shown to be wildly over-optimistic.

Most forecasters agree that mental illness will become an increasingly important problem. The evidence we already have supports such a suggestion. In 1970 in the United States of America an average of one prescription for a psychotropic drug was written and dispensed for every member of the American population. The cost of all these drugs amounted to approximately one thousand million dollars. According to *Health in 1980-90. A predictive study based on an international inquiry* by Philip Selby, `Surveys have shown that one adult American out of four takes at least one psychotropic drug regularly, while over half the population uses them from time to time.' All the evidence points to the increase in the consumption of drugs with an inevitable increase in the incidence of side effects and the problem of habituation and addiction.

There are already many hundreds of thousands of people addicted to or dependent upon the drugs prescribed for them by doctors. The drug-dependent population greatly exceeds the population of alcohol or hard-drug users. Dealing with these people is going to be a major problem which will surely produce a variety of possible solutions.

The future could, for example, bring many useful advances in the electronic control of the human brain. Already doctors have learned how to stimulate the brain electronically and control the activities of patients. Such a technique might well be useful and valuable if all doctors were totally honourable men and unlikely to be seduced by power and money. Unfortunately, doctors are all too human and can easily be seduced by both.

It would be quite possible to control the behaviour of people very effectively with electrodes implanted in the brain. Such controlled citizens would be cheaper to build and run than robots and would have the tremendous advantage of being self-duplicating. It would not be difficult to sell the idea of electronic stimulation of the brain to people seduced by the offers of pleasure' at the 'touch of a button'. Indeed, many would probably pay for the privilege of being turned into human tools. Many of those dependent on psychotropic drugs would accept the offer or at least agree if their supply of drugs were threatened. From there it would be a short step to the implantation of more electrodes to control other emotions and thought processes. Workers required for humble tasks could be given a large number of electrodes so that their every movement was controlled and workers expected to think a little for themselves could perhaps have fewer implanted electrodes.

Doctors working in the field of human genetics may well in the future have a tremendous influence on the type of lives we lead. Activities in this area have already had far-reaching elects and medical progress has adversely affected the genetic quality of the human race. The incidence of curable genetic disorders will continue to rise, thereby putting an increasingly intolerable strain on the resources of the health services of the world, and ensuring that the population contains an increasing proportion of people unable to work and live normally.

If the quality of life is not to deteriorate too much, we will have to accept one or other of the methods of control offered by the researchers in the field of genetics. We have little choice about whether we do something or not; the decision has been forced upon us by the advances which have been made, and our choice simply involves the way in which we deal with the problem.

None of the possibilities is attractive. Well-meaning but uninformed people concerned about the rights of the individual have vehemently opposed attempts to sterilise those who are mentally or physically disabled and who will pass those traits on to their children. Those opposing compulsory sterilisation argue, quite reasonably, that even a mentally retarded human being should have the right to decide for herself whether or not she will have children. And anyway, who is to decide who is mentally retarded?

It cannot be disputed that such an argument is a reasonable and humane one. The difficulty is, I am afraid, that if we act in a reasonable and humane way, our future is a very bleak one. The world could, in a few generations' time, be largely populated by the insane and the physically disabled, and even the most reasonable and humane people have to admit that the insane and physically disabled would live uncomfortable lives without a reasonable population of sane and physically capable people to look after them.

Will the protests of the anti-abortion brigade be ignored and will therapeutic abortions be offered to women carrying deformed babies? We do not yet know what the true risks of ultrasound and amniocentesis are, and there will undoubtedly be many who will argue that the woman who has a therapeutic abortion because she is carrying a malformed child will suffer badly.

Or will genetic surgery develop as another speciality within medicine and will genetic surgeons operate to ensure that only perfect babies are born? It is possible to freeze sperm and keep it for years. It is possible for a woman to choose the sex of her baby. It is possible to keep an animal's head alive without its body. It is possible to produce mice which can breathe under water. Research has been done which enables doctors to move patients about from afar by pushing buttons which fire impulses into the brain. Psychosurgery has been done on disobedient children to turn them into obedient children. Work on artificial eyes which work like television cameras is progressing fast. How long will it be before genetic surgeons can Xerox human beings? And when commercial laboratories and money-hungry Harley Street doctors get hold of such techniques, what will happen? How long will it be before superman has the legs of a kangaroo, the nose of a bloodhound, the ears of a dog, the eyes of a hawk, the arms of a gorilla, the brain of a Nobel prize-winner, the sonar of a bat, the strength of a bear and the beauty of an Adonis? Or will we merely be content to breed a race of identically perfect men and women, distinguishable from one another only by numbers tattooed on their wrists?

Another result of the work done by medical researchers will be that many more elderly and infirm people will be alive. Already the number of old people alive is increasing at a tremendous rate. The burden on the younger generations is becoming more and more intolerable. With the virtual break down of the family unit, the result is that hospitals and old peoples' homes have very long waiting lists. There has been comparatively little work done to find out how best the elderly can be kept alive and independent; the work which has been done has been designed rather to keep the elderly and dependent alive. Research workers only seem interested in the moribund.

The difficulties will grow. The number of old people living to their eighties and nineties will increase as the population grows. Even if average life expectation is falling, the falling birth rate, the increasing population and the decrease in infant mortalities will mean that the average age of the population increases. The number of old people to be looked after, by a shrinking number of others, will expand at an uncontrollable rate. If those old people are not taught how to look after themselves, and after one another, there will be only one horrifying and frightening alternative.

Euthanasia already has a number of proponents. A number of doctors believe that it is the only answer to the problem of what to do with the aged. There are, of course, several types of euthanasia. There is the problem of what to do with the dying and dependent patient who will never be independent again but who can be saved temporarily by medical knowledge, and there is the problem of what to do with the fit but dependent old person who is not dying and who will never be independent again. Many doctors already practice a type of euthanasia on patients in the first group. I myself believe it is sometimes realistic, kind and humane to allow a dying patient to die in dignity.

But what do we do with the patients in the second group? What do we do with those who are incontinent, mentally confused, physically dependent but likely to live for another five or ten years?

When the number of such patients is relatively small, we can provide nursing care for them (though we do so with difficulty already) but what happens when the numbers continue to grow, as they surely will? Then the only alternatives will be either to send the disabled old people back into the homes of their younger relatives, allowing many of them to die un-nursed and uncared for or to provide them with a clean and peaceful medical death.

Medical progress is pushing us slowly but certainly towards this choice. The only other alternative is to divert our research resources towards finding better ways of helping the elderly to care for themselves, towards the development of better aids and equipment and towards the development of screening programmes and health education programmes designed to help the elderly to maintain themselves in better physical condition.

As well as these additional problems, the problems we already have will still be with us. And of these perhaps one of the most worrying is the problem of how to choose whom to treat. We simply cannot treat all the patients who need treatment. We could not treat every patient to the best of our ability if we spent every single penny we all earned on medical care. If we abandoned our defence programme, our housing programmes, our educational programmes, our cultural programmes, our sporting programmes and so on, we would still not be able to provide surgical care and kidney dialysis for every patient who wanted it. Even in Britain, only a proportion of the patients who could be saved by kidney dialysis would be saved if we pumped all our National Health Service resources into this one aspect of medical care, involving a comparatively small number of patients.

Treatment programmes are costing more and more. It costs a great deal of money to perform an open heart operation, for example, and so surgeons have to be selective. They choose the patients whom they think will do best. But what right has a surgeon to decide whose life is worth saving? These ethical problems are getting worse and worse rather than better and better. The cost of complex equipment is rising, the number of staff involved in a single operation is increasing, the number of people needing the operation is rising and the percentage of disappointed patients who must be left to die unless they can save the necessary money is also rising. The newspapers are always carrying stories of unhappy mothers whose children will die because they cannot have such and such an operation. The lucky ones who receive the most publicity will live because the public will give them money to hire private surgeons and private treatment.

As much as we may wish to treat the sick and the dying, we must learn to understand that we have at least reached a time when it is not always possible to do so. Priorities have to be selected; some patients have to be left to die; some diseases which have interested politically powerful people will receive unreasonable amounts of money and other diseases which are politically unfashionable will receive little attention. It is my belief that it would be infinitely fairer to spend our valuable resources on preventing sickness rather than on struggling to improve our temporary solutions, when those temporary solutions will at best provide relief for a small proportion of sufferers.

What sort of additional problems is the future likely to bring? Judging the speed of change in medicine is rather like trying to predict the height of waves in the sea. If the wind blows from one direction, the waves can be judged with some certainty. If, however, the wind changes and waves come from another direction, there will be interference between wave trains and peaks may summate or waves may disappear altogether. New developments can change the whole scene.

The immediate problems of fertility control, food preservation, environmental pollution, overpopulation, organ transplantation, neurosurgery, computerised medicine, artificial organs and the therapeutic manipulation of genes seem enough to be going on with. Artificial hearts and artificial lungs will lead to ethical, social and economic problems dwarfing those of the artificial kidney. It is already possible to tell the sex of a foetus from amniocentesis and it may soon be possible to kill off specific sperm types in the vagina with the aid of a simple douche, so creating a baby of specific sex. What will industry make of these possibilities? How will sperm banks advertise in the future when they are allowed to buy television space? What is the future of the general practitioner who, we are assured will soon have a blood and urine analyser in his little black bag? How long will we be allowed to go around polluting everyone else's atmosphere with our cigarettes and motor cars? Should foetuses which carry genes which suggest that the final result will be a criminal be dragged off to police abortoirs? What will they put in our water after fluoride?

These are all problems which already exist and they are problems which we have not even started to try to solve.

As to the distant future, surely nothing is now impossible. Arthur C. Clarke has written that 'When a distinguished but elderly scientist states that something is impossible he is very probably wrong.' Clarke, incidentally, defines an elderly scientist as one over the age of 30. Clarke's third law is that 'Any sufficiently advanced technology is indistinguishable from magic'.

Those who practise medicine and understand computers and other electronic aids believe sincerely that machines – that is to say, robots – will soon be built which can do everything that a man can do. Everything. One American company has announced a new memory device which could store inside a six-foot cube all the information recorded during the last 10,000 years. Machines will be able to design and build bigger and better and brighter machines which are self-repairing and self-reproducing. The general principles underlying the construction of such machines have already been worked out. Machines already exist which can learn by experience. They would undoubtedly be better suited to underwater exploration and space travel.

There are literally no limits to the possibilities. It was difficult enough to see what problems our discoveries would produce when inventions as comparatively simple and uncomplicated as the motor car were first introduced. In the 'Scientific American' in 1899 there was a discussion on the possible effects of the motor car on city life and one participant is reputed to have stated that the motor car would help improve our cities in many ways. He saw cities with clean streets, without dust or smells, and swift and noiseless vehicles eliminating the strain and distractions of city life.

I hope that my forecasts and fears will prove to be unreasonably pessimistic but I do not believe that they will. Our only real hope is to do something now about the problems we already have, to spend much more effort on trying to protect ourselves from our own discoveries; to spend far less time and effort on traditional research and far more time and effort on more practical problems.

12. The Environment

This book will undoubtedly attract a number of critics from among the great population of research workers. The traditional reply to those who attack research programmes of any kind is to accuse the attacker of having no compassion, and of having no interest in the saving of human life. This is an easy argument to put forward. A representative of some of the companies manufacturing patent medicines once accused me of a lack of humanity when I attacked his companies for the irresponsible promotion of ineffective but dangerous medicines.

To forestall this response and to avoid the criticism that I have written a destructive account of medical research which contains no guidance for the future, I shall in the next part of the book write at some length about the work which could be done if we had the money and workers to do it. I shall, in this and the next two chapters, describe in detail the problems which do need elucidation, the research programmes which do need initiating, the techniques which do need assessing, and the areas of preventive medicine where relatively small amounts of money spent could result in relatively large savings in human life.

It is my contention that those involved in medical research programmes often have little understanding of the real needs of the community at large but are too concerned with their own glorification. This is a serious accusation but one which I think is realistic. It is an unfortunate fact that we just cannot afford to do everything we want to do. We cannot afford to treat all the people who need treating, we cannot afford to save all the lives we could save. It is my belief that we should spend what resources we have as wisely as we can and do what we can to improve the quality and quantity of life for every citizen.

The tremendous improvement in life expectation which occurred during the nineteenth century was due to the improvement in environmental conditions. Sadly, this century has seen a steady deterioration again in the quality of the environment and this deterioration is undoubtedly responsible for much of the illness and many of the early deaths which still plague us. A greater general understanding of the pollutants responsible for ill health and the ways in which those pollutants could be eradicated or controlled would without doubt contribute greatly to the eradication and control of much sickness. This chapter deals with environmental problems.

It took 1700 years, from the year 1 to the year 1700, for the world population to double. The next doubling took from 1700 to 1850 and the present world population of about 4,000 million will, it is estimated, double in the next 35 years. One result of this massive increase in the world's population is a similar increase in the amount of waste produced. In Britain 2 pounds of dry refuse per person are collected and tipped daily. In America the figure is 4 pounds. A total of about 5 million cubic metres of domestic sewage and 3 million cubic metres of industrial waste are discharged daily along the south and east coasts of Britain, together with 7 million cubic metres of cooling water from power stations. About 10 million tons of industrial waste are tipped each year, half a million tons being toxic or acidic.

Advances in technology add daily to the environmental hazards. Radioactive and petroleum wastes contaminate water, earth and air. Motor cars and factories pour out enormous quantities of potentially poisonous substances. About 2,000 cases of lead poisoning were reported in slum neighbourhoods of Chicago in one recent year. Fourteen youngsters died and 40 per cent of the rest suffered some neurological damage or some mental retardation. Very little research has been done into the scale of environmental pollution and the effects the pollutants are likely to have upon the human race.

Our atmosphere is heavily polluted with carbon monoxide, sulphur compounds, pesticides, mercury, lead, asbestos and countless other potentially toxic and mutagenic substances which can be absorbed by an exposed person without him being aware of their presence in his environment. This is the real danger with environmental pollutants. They diminish the quality of life but they do it so slowly and insidiously that the victim does not complain. In a Mexican village recently it was found that local peasants had got accustomed to drinking water which contained large quantities of arsenic. In Britain hundreds of thousands of men and women have chronic chest conditions which are sometimes caused and always exacerbated by the air they breathe. Thousands of factory workers who have worked in noisy factories have impaired hearing as do many who live near busy motorways and airports. Few complain about pollutants which take half a lifetime to act.

Environmental pollutants which do not cause any apparent ill-effects under normal conditions can become dangerous under stressful conditions. For example, lead which is stored in the bones may be released into the circulation during an attack of pneumonia. Pesticides and toxic substances can be stored in the liver or body fats and released during infective, emotional or physiological stress episodes. According to René Dubos, `Many different kinds of physiological or infectious stresses can act as triggers to activate potential toxicities that would otherwise remain unmanifested under usual conditions'.

We all know that air pollutants can cause disease. The effects of smoke on the lungs are well documented. But not everyone knows that researchers have shown that particles taken from our air have increased the incidence of tumour formation in mice. There is no immediate relationship – the tumours form in an adult mouse if as a new-born mouse it is brought into contact with the particles. It may well be that babies living in badly polluted areas are breathing in dangerous materials which may cause tumours in later life. We just do not know because the air has not been polluted for long enough.

Steady and loud noises can cause irreversible damage and workers whose hearing has been damaged by exposure to heavy noises at work can claim damages in many countries. American courts have awarded large amounts of compensation to such victims. Experiments have shown that the heart rate of the foetus can be accelerated by noises to which the mother makes no reaction. The sonic boom produced by such aeroplanes as Concorde may cause irreversible physiological damage as well as mental damage. Our environment is persistently polluted in many ways and there have been few scientific studies of the long-term effects of the pollutants. It has taken two decades to establish the statistical relationship between smoking cigarettes and developing lung cancer. Many similar relationships may exist. Could it be, for example, that industrial wastes and waste gases from automobile exhaust systems are related to the increasing incidence of heart attacks? If so, surely it is better to catch the pyromaniac than to rush around trying to extinguish the blazes after he has started them.

One of the particular problems of environmental pollutants is that they do not produce useful genetic changes. The victim's descendants will be just as susceptible as was the victim. Those suffering from chronic bronchitis breed before developing the disease. There is no chance at all that the human body will ever adapt to cope with the pollutants in the environment.

If it were only the external environment which were polluted, it would theoretically be possible for man to protect himself by building sound-proofed homes with effective air-conditioning. Unfortunately, however, factories and offices commonly expose workers to conditions which are unpleasant and potentially dangerous. For some unknown reason, trade unionists who will complain so bitterly about a cut in the length of their tea break or the loss of some minor privilege, will apparently happily ignore the fact that they are all being slowly poisoned to death. New substances and new techniques are being introduced into factories and offices so quickly and in such numbers that there is no chance to evaluate potential health dangers before large numbers of people have been affected. Even then the pollutants go unchecked, for there are few if any factories where checks are kept on the health of the working population and where there is any chance of detecting evidence of pathological changes before they are irreversible and untreatable.

In a report of a WHO study group in 1975 entitled 'Early Detection of Health Impairment in Occupational Exposure to Health Hazards', a number of examples of substances which cause respiratory impairment are named. These include mineral fibrogenic dusts such as silicon dioxide, chemical agents such as beryllium, biological agents such as enzyme washing powders, and vegetable dusts such as those found in the air in food-processing factories, textile factories and agricultural industries.

The writers of the WHO report pointed out that 'For many physic-chemical work factors adequate exposure effect response relationships in human beings are not known; many permissible limits are based mainly on animal data, not evaluated in epidemiological studies.

The report went on `...it is not known whether there are any quantitative relationships between medium noise levels and presbyacusis; whether noise leads to social alienation; whether long-term exposure to solvents affects brain function; or whether cardiovascular health is impaired by exposure to carbon monoxide or to various metals' and concluded, 'There is a pressing need for research to elaborate simple and practical diagnostic methods for use in occupational health practice for the early detection of health impairment and exposure.'

One cannot be surprised at the indifference of the working population to the health hazards they are exposed to when one considers the continued success of the tobacco companies in selling their lethal products. Cigarettes are now known to cause lung cancer, cancer of the mouth, cancer of the larynx, bronchitis, emphysema, ischaemic heart disease, cerebrovascular diseases, peptic ulceration of the stomach, underweight babies and many psychological problems. This list is taken from a World Health Organisation publication, 'Smoking and its Effects on Health', published in 1975.

Cigarettes cause one-third of all cancer deaths in Britain; children of those who smoke have increased tendency to have respiratory diseases and those who have asthma and other allergic conditions often suffer badly as a result of exposure to cigarette smoke. As the WHO put it, 'Children of parents who smoke are not only at risk before they are born but suffer an increased risk of potentially serious illness during their first year of life'.

Despite this evidence, opposed only by a few eccentrics working for the tobacco companies, the medical profession has been slow to take a stand and oppose the sale of tobacco. The vast majority of doctors have themselves stopped smoking but the official medical organisations have refused to get involved. According to Greenberg in *The Quality of Care* ... few of the AMA's stands have been more disgraceful than its action a few years ago when it accepted a ten million dollar research grant from six tobacco companies (after publication of a Government report on the overwhelming evidence of the insidious effects of smoking on health) and came out against placing a warning label on cigarette packages.' Much tobacco company money has found its way into research centres in Britain too. Surveys have shown that although by far the most effective way of stopping patients from smoking is for a doctor to advise them to do so, this rarely happens. Three-quarters of all smokers express a desire to stop but less than a quarter succeed in doing this. If advised by a doctor to stop smoking, over a third succeed permanently.

Even if you lived in a sound-proof house and had an efficient air-conditioner and drank only distilled water, you would still be exposed to a steady attack by pollutants as long as you continued to eat. For several decades now, food prices have been kept down by bulk production and by packaging and marketing techniques which often involve the use of chemicals. Some additives are used to disguise inferior tasteless foods, others to aid mass production, some to boost the size of the product. Some additives are added to the product while it is still growing, others are added during preparation, and yet more added as preservatives. Whether packaged or allegedly fresh, food-stuffs on sale today are almost certainly contaminated. We must not forget that on top of deliberate adulteration, there is also much accidental contamination, caused by environmental pollutants carried into the soil by a rainstorm or into an animal through its food.

In 1955 a joint meeting of the Food and Agricultural Organisation of the United Nations and the World Health Organisation began vetting food additives for safety. In the case of chemicals an acceptable daily intake (ADI) was decided upon; this usually being one hundredth of the level found to be just without toxic effect in the species of animal most susceptible to its toxic activity. Only in 1974 did the FAO and the WHO recommend that ADIs should take into account the amount of naturally occurring chemicals as well as added chemicals. It is still not possible to assess the potential cumulative effects of chemicals consumed, nor do we know what happens when chemicals mix in the body.

Early adulteration of foods was quite horrifying, with enormous amounts of mercury, lead and arsenic being used. These substances are still in use. Preservatives, colourings, sweeteners and pesticide residues mix with hormones and antibiotics used as animal feed additives. In 1967 it was estimated that the consumption of food additives in the USA was running at 3.5 kilos per head per year. According to the WHO 'Chronicle' in 1970, 'In the last decade the use of food additives (and even more of pesticides) has grown on an almost geometric scale. Internationally accepted rules for their use are an urgent necessity.' And it is still getting worse. As a leader writer in the *British Medical Journal* pointed out in February 1975, 'Only a fine line separates the use of chemicals for these reasons [preservation and processing] and the unnecessary adulteration of food for no reason other than profit.' For example, most of the colours added are without nutritive value but are added to make the food sell. The 1974 FAO/WHO meeting considered 29 food colourings used. For only six of these was there enough information to establish ADIs. The others were used, although neither the authorities nor the manufacturers knew what the effects would be on the consumers. There are about 3,000 different additives used altogether. Half of these add colour or flavour.

The pollution of food goes on outside the factories and packing sheds of course. Water polluted with mercury discharged as factory wastes can mean that fish caught there contain dangerous amounts of mercury. Lead compounds used as petrol additives also contaminate foods since the fall-out from vehicle exhausts often collects on food crops. Lead is a cumulative poison which can enter the body either by inhalation or by ingestion. ingestion. Lead can cause permanent brain damage and mental retardation, and in some urban areas in Britain over 5 per cent of all children have high blood lead levels. Doctors merely 'tut tut' and society arranges for more schools for the educationally subnormal.

The consumption of drugs has also reached a frightening level. Relatively few researchers are involved in studies to determine the carcinogenic or other toxic effects of drugs. We know little about the reactions of the human body to the long-term ingestion of pain killers, hormone pills, tranquillisers and so on. The addition of antibiotics to animal foodstuffs means that even the healthy receive their steady supply of drugs.

Drug companies and even academic research centres are at present primarily concerned in the search for new drugs to replace old ones or to fill gaps in the therapeutic armoury. Little research is done into the packaging of drugs, the tailoring of doses to suit individual patients, the development of new methods of administration and the problems of addiction and habituation. Another problem frequently ignored is the fact that supplies of ingredients for drugs are in increasingly short supply. According to the representative of one major company, `Effort and technical ingenuity must be directed from the search for new drugs in order to maintain the supply of existing remedies.'

Ten per cent of all hospital admissions (a total of 507,000 in the United Kingdom) are originally due to accidents or poisonings.

According to the `Medical Annual' for 1975, one-fifth of these were due to accidents in the home and 17 per cent were due to road accidents. Expenditure on research into the cause of accidents is low, although, as Dr H. Mahler, Director General of the World Health Organisation pointed out in the Inaugural Lecture of the British Postgraduate Medical Federation's 1975/6 series of lectures on the Scientific Basis of Medicine in London in October 1975, it is more sensible for a city burns unit which has been kept busy dealing with injuries caused by scalding coffee to redesign the faulty coffee pot responsible for the burns than to research into more effective ways of treating burns.

I would add finally that the number of people killed on our roads makes it reasonable to describe automobile accidents as having reached epidemic proportions. It is surely the responsibility of the medical profession to help reduce the number of deaths and injuries related to automobile accidents. According to the magazine *World Health*, 'If traffic accidents are tackled by methods similar to those used against the great killing diseases, the present epidemic of road deaths could be brought under control like plague and smallpox.'

13. Medical Practices

One of the reasons why doctors are currently on the defensive, protecting themselves against attacks from outside the profession, is that there is good evidence to show that much of modern medical practice detracts from the quality of life rather than adding to it. There is strong evidence to show that doctors themselves cause a great deal of suffering and that a society can suffer just as much from a surfeit of medical care as it can from a shortage. In the past doctors have defended quite fiercely their right to practise totally independently, without any sort of outside assessment or interference. The time has now come when doctors will have to learn to assess their own practices as well as the drugs they use. They will have to be more self-critical and ensure that – as Hippocrates is said to have suggested – they `first do no harm'. This chapter contains a discussion of some of the specific problems which need consideration and research; problems which can be divided into two main categories, dealing with either the waste involved in modern medical practices or the damage done by doctors to their patients. Medical wastages are discussed first.

Despite the enormous amounts of money spent on research, little if any is spent on finding out whether or not medical procedures are effective, why doctors' prescribing habits vary so much and why there are so many fashions in a supposedly scientific profession. The tradition of clinical freedom means that doctors can ignore advice based on established medical practice, ignore the needs of the patients and simply do what they want to do.

There have always been fashions in medicine. In seventeenth-century France Louis XIII had 212 enemas, 215 purges and 47 bleedings in a single year. The Canon of Troyes is reputed to have had a total of 2190 enemas in a two-year period. Today there are many fashions but the removal of tonsils is perhaps one of the longest-lasting and most enduring. Tonsils were removed from between a half and three-quarters of all children in the 1930s. This often useless and unnecessary, and always potentially hazardous operation is the one most commonly performed in the United States.

About 1,100.000 such operations are done there each year. Between 200 and 300 deaths a year are caused by the operation for the removal of tonsils. Few of those would have died from tonsillitis!

The American Child Health Association conducted an unusual survey a few years ago. They surveyed 1000 children of 11 years in New York. Of these 61 per cent had had their tonsils out when first seen. The remaining 39 per cent were then referred to physicians, who recommended that about half had their tonsils out. And so it went on, until only 65 pairs of tonsils remained uncondemned. The study then stopped because the Child Health Association ran out of doctors to consult.

Appendicitis is another fashionable operation. One German study suggested that the German mortality rate from appendicitis is three times higher than in any other country, simply because appendicectomies are performed three times as often in Germany as anywhere else. A follow up of 959 deaths showed that only 1 in 4 patients actually had acute appendicitis at the time of their operation. The other 719 had at least died fashionably.

New medical ideas are often accepted readily by people on the lookout for death-defying disease interceptors. A technique or method which works sometimes will eventually become a routine. According to Henry Miller, whose views I do not always share, 'Medicine is to a striking degree dominated by a succession of fashions. At the present time everything is due to a disturbance of immune mechanisms.' Among routines fondly favoured by doctors are such things as intravenous therapy. A century or two ago doctors spent much of their time busily removing blood from their patients. Bleeding was a most popular form of treatment for just about everything. Today doctors spend much of their time busily putting things into their patients' bloodstreams.

Laboratory tests are also a fashionable part of modern medical practice. Most doctors are trained to use the laboratory as a crutch. They use it to help them make a diagnosis which could just as effectively be made without the laboratory. For example, tests are done when the diagnosis has been made on clinical grounds, just to provide laboratory support. The result is that the number of laboratory tests done each year is rising dramatically. According to Professor Vincent Marks, Professor of Clinical Biochemistry at the University of Surrey, quoted in *General Practitioner* on 5 September

1975, the number of biochemical tests done in Britain represents an average of one a year for every man, woman and child. Professor Marks believes that most of these tests have no value. Other experts have shown that the number of tests done is growing at a rate of about 15 per cent per year. Few clinicians are as brave as the consultant physician in London who said, 'If the clinical observation and the laboratory findings are incompatible, the laboratory findings are wrong.' Most doctors believe the laboratory first and the patient second.

The value of laboratory investigations was put into perspective by Doctors Hampton, Mitchell, Harrison, Prichard and Seymour, writing in the *British Medical Journal* on 31 May 1975. In an article entitled 'The relative contributions of history taking, physical examination and laboratory investigations to diagnosis and management of medical out-patients' they concluded that 'A diagnosis that agreed with the one finally accepted was made after reading the referral letter and taking the history in 66 out of 80 new patients; the physical examination was useful in only 7 patients, and the laboratory investigations in a further 7. In only 1 out of 6 patients in whom the physician was unable to make any diagnosis after taking the history and examining the patient did laboratory investigations lead to a positive diagnosis.'

The length of time a patient stays in hospital is also very variable for no good reason. In a book entitled *Rationing Health Care*, Michael Cooper quotes a study which found that the removal of tonsils and adenoids resulted in a six-day hospital stay for over 80 per cent of cases at one hospital but in a stay of only one day in another hospital for over half of the cases.

Dr Robert Logan of Manchester University has estimated that if the British national average of 12-day stays in hospital were cut to the nine days some regions have achieved hospital waiting lists could be cleared within a year. The national average stay for hernia patients is 11 days, while some hospitals average 21 days. A study published in *The Lancet* in 1968 said that patients discharged after seven days suffered no ill effects. But still no one has done any research to find out which consultants are keeping patients in hospital unnecessarily, and to find out why some consultants take patients into hospital to do tests which could be performed on out-patients. It has been estimated that up to one third of all patients in

American and British hospitals do not need to be there and that if the average length of stay in hospital in America could be cut by a single day it would produce a saving of more than 1.7 billion dollars a year.

Wastage and bad practice are unfortunately common in most countries. In an article entitled 'Rationalising requests for X ray films in neurology' published in the *BMJ* in 1968 by Dr Bull and Dr Zilkha, it was pointed out that very many X ray pictures are taken for no really good reason but done merely as thoughtless routine which no one has bothered to question.

We need to look more carefully into the reasons why certain types of operations are performed. Operations for varicose veins, for example are sometimes done for cosmetic reasons. In other words, the operation is done not because the varicose veins are causing any medical problems but because they make the legs unsightly. Is this a problem which we should be treating in a time when the NHS cannot afford to treat all of its patients? It is difficult to select areas to ignore but we have to do this; in particular, we often have to select patients to ignore. One of the most common problems aired in public is the cost of treating patients on hospital dialysis. It now costs about £8,000 a year to look after a patient needing dialysis in hospital (that does not include the initial cost of the equipment and the buildings) and there are about 5,000 patients a year who would benefit from such treatment. That means that on artificial kidneys alone we could easily be spending £40,000,000 each year. That sum would be increased in each succeeding year as more and more patients in kidney failure required treatment.

A paper published in the *British Journal of Preventive and Social Medicine* in August 1971, entitled 'Expected and observed values for the prescription of Vitamin B12 in England and Wales' and written by A.L.Cochrane and F.Moore, provided a sad commentary on the prescribing habits of doctors. The authors chose the prescribing of Vitamin B12 since the drug involved is practically specific for one condition and since there are accepted standard therapeutic doses. In other words it should have been possible to calculate accurately the amount of Vitamin B12 prescribed from a knowledge of the incidence of the disease concerned. In actual fact the researchers found that the ratio between the observed and expected consumption of Vitamin B12 was as high as 20 to 1.

In 1951 a report of the Central Midwives Board stated that the discharge of patients before the tenth day after delivery is 'an undesirable practice'. In 1953 the Ministry of Health issued a circular stating that 'maternity patients should not be discharged before the tenth day'. More recently research has shown that 48-hour stays are usually quite long enough. Indeed, as Dr Donald Gould pointed out in the 'New Statesman' on 12 September 1975, Holland has a lower infant mortality rate than Britain and a lower maternal mortality rate too and yet two-thirds of Dutch women have their babies at home, whereas in Britain a great deal of money has been spent on providing facilities for women to have their babies in hospital. Giving birth used to be a fairly simple process. Today it involves ultrasound, amniocentesis, epidural anaesthesia, pelvic arteriography and a dozen other complicated, expensive and dangerous procedures.

Operating techniques have improved enormously in the last half of the century and it is now comparatively safe to have an operation. There are, however, still measurable risks and in the United Kingdom alone surgical deaths are said to number between 20,000 and 30,000 a year. Many of the conditions which took these patients into the operating theatres might not have proved fatal by themselves.

One recent study showed that 'the mortality risk of elective herniorrhaphy in a population of men over 65 years was four times greater than the risk of allowing strangulation to occur in a minority and then having to perform emergency surgery. This simply means that if you are a 66-year-old man and you have a hernia, it may well be safer for you to keep your hernia and have it operated upon only if it causes pain and needs emergency attention.

A great deal of money in Britain and in other Western countries is spent on the provision and running of intensive care units. Most medium-sized or large hospitals now have these small wards which contain the latest equipment and which are staffed by highly trained doctors and nurses. Patients recovering from surgery or from heart attacks are usually nursed in these units for a short period. There is, however, evidence which suggests that patients may not benefit at all from having a bed in such a unit and that indeed, on the contrary, they may suffer.

Patients who have had heart attacks are very often put into one of these units where the costs run as high as £500 a week. However, those with open minds are now questioning the point of it all. According to an anaesthetist at St Thomas's Hospital in London, in no more than 10 per cent of cases can one say that being in an ITU has saved a life.

A report published in the *British Medical Journal* in August 1971 entitled 'Acute Myocardial Infarction: home and hospital treatment' included a study of 1,203 patients with heart attacks. The patients concerned were allocated at random to either a hospital bed or a bed in their own homes. The authors of the paper concluded 'The mortality rates of the random groups are similar for home and hospital treatment'.

Speaking at a conference in Winchester in October 1974, Dr R. Wood, a consultant physician, pointed out that the reason why patients in coronary care units may do better than patients in other hospital wards or at home is simply because in these units defibrillators are available. These are by no means machines which can only be used in coronary care units though they are usually used most in such units simply because they are stored there. Dr Wood suggested that the other expensive equipment may be irrelevant. The defibrillator could just as easily be stored in a ward sluice.

According to Michael Cooper in *Rationing Health Care*, there is a growing body of evidence that much medical practice is, if not unsound, then at least unproven. Large-scale cancer surgery, insulin treatment for diabetes, tonsillectomy, and hospital bed rest for both coronary heart disease and tuberculosis are some examples which have been examined and found wanting. Nine out of ten surgical operations are done to improve life rather than save life but little research has ever been done to find out if all those operations actually do improve the quality of life.'

Surgery for small-cell cancer of the bronchus has been shown by some controlled trials to lessen rather than to lengthen the life expectancy of the patient concerned. And while excessive tonsillectomies are being performed, children in Liverpool and the surrounding area who need open heart surgery are having to wait up to three years, with the result that they deteriorate so much that the final outcome of the operation is affected. We have, sadly, to remember that the leech bottle managed to survive after the First World War in some British hospitals and ask how many of our modern techniques are equally out of date and pointless. Very little research has been done to find out just what is useful and what is not in modern medical practice. Many of our customs and habits have never been proved to be worthwhile. For example, dealing with dental disease costs millions of pounds every year but there is little or no evidence to show that this is all money well spent. Over half of all Britons over the age of 45 have lost all their teeth. There is no evidence to show, for example, that school dental care does any good at all. The money might well be better spent on giving away apples to schoolchildren.

Even some fashionable types of preventive medicine are expensive and non-productive. Screening programmes are considered by many to be the solution to a number of our medical problems and to offer an effective way of improving our mortality and morbidity figures. The problems involved in organising such a screening programme are well illustrated by the difficulties in organising a breast cancer screening campaign. Any screening programme must satisfy a number of criteria: it must be fairly cheap and easy to run; it must enable doctors to pick up, at an early stage, a treatable condition; it must not be dangerous or harmful to those who do not have the disease, and so on. Many powerful lobbyists have argued that breast cancer screening should be available to all women. Doctors with great experience of this particular area of medicine say, however, that breast screening programmes do not prove very effective and are certainly not economical. They involve highly trained staff in a great deal of work and unless special 'at risk' groups of women are selected, the number of women with treatable breast cancers is very small.

The size of the problem can be seen from the fact that there are approximately 20 million pairs of breasts in the United Kingdom. Those who support the idea that breast screening programmes should be made available to all women may not realise it, but this means that if every woman had her breasts examined once a year and each surgeon involved (the person doing the examining has got to be very skilled) can examine 50 women a day then 2,000 surgeons will be involved in doing nothing but simply look for lumps. There would not be any surgeons left to get on with removing lumps which felt cancerous.

Selecting women in 'at risk' groups to have their breasts examined is difficult because those selected worry (they know they have been considered 'at risk') and those not selected also worry (they see their friends being examined and wonder why they can't be given the 'all clear').

Screening for cervical cancer is also of doubtful value. According to AL. Cochrane in *Effectiveness and Efficiency*, 'The death rate from carcinoma of the cervix was falling before smears were introduced and has continued to fall at roughly the same rate in most areas.' Cochrane's point is that we may well spend millions of pounds on cervical screening campaigns when in fact these screening programmes are having no real effect on the incidence of the disease and the survival rate of women with the disease.

Similar problems arise when one considers screening for chest conditions, screening for diabetes, hypertension and so on. All of these conditions need spotting at an early stage if morbidity levels are to be reduced but screening programmes must involve highly trained staff. Commercial organisations which provide screening services charge considerable sums for fairly basic tests. Many experts believe that, done badly, screening programmes such as the cervical screening programmes are a waste of time and money and that done well they would cost far more than we could afford. The point is that if we had lifeguards stationed every 200 yards along every inland waterway, we would undoubtedly be able to prevent many drowning accidents. It would, unfortunately, be an expensive method of preventing accidents, nevertheless the mothers of the children saved each year would consider it a very worthwhile expense.

It may well be that there are far more productive (though less fashionable) areas for screening programmes than breast cancer and cervical cancer. According to the Scottish geriatrician, Sir Ferguson Anderson, there is an enormous amount of undetectable illness among many old people and old people are often reluctant to report their illness to anyone. It is certainly true that home accidents are common among the weakened elderly, that putting an old person into hospital is very costly and often inhumane and that the number of old people in the community is growing at a tremendous rate. It is also known that health visitors and district nurses can keep an eye on relatively large numbers of old people at relatively low expense. Such a screening programme would not be fashionable but would probably be cost-effective and productive.

Despite their willingness to experiment with new techniques and new equipment, doctors are extraordinarily slow to adopt new methods of administration which might help improve the quality of the service they provide. There has been a great deal of half-hearted research into such problems as how to store medical records and make them more easily readable and available but doctors are dreadful reactionaries when experimenting that close to home. General practitioners in Britain, for example, are likely to change from a small record folder to a large one in the next few years. Their representatives seem to have totally ignored the possibility of using microfilm as a storage medium.

In thousands of hospitals and health centres and doctors' surgeries patients' records are in absolute chaos. Millions of folders are stored in huge dusty rooms where they are difficult to find at the best of times and impossible to get hold of in a hurry. The folders all contain much information which is totally irrelevant but which is kept because of a tradition that all information should be stored. There is, so the theory goes; always the chance that someone may want to know how Mr Wilson slept on 18 May 1946 or how many times Mrs Roberts had her bowels open on 9 March 1941.

The result is that hospitals have to employ people just to look after the notes and if the one set available is lost, there is no replacement. A filing expert who recently did some research for one large London hospital estimated that one per cent of the patients' records are lost every year. In the hospital he studied 12 people were employed to do nothing but look for lost notes. That same hospital stored notes for half a million patients several miles away and the files were growing at a rate of 100,000 new patients a year. When the record clerks are off duty (two-thirds of the time) the notes are completely unavailable.

Computers have been suggested as a method of storing data but there are many problems. For one thing it is difficult to store the doctor's notes as he wrote them; for another it is difficult to ensure that the notes are permanently available without specialist help or expensive equipment. Thirdly, there is the problem that computer-stored information is relatively easy to get hold of. There is, therefore, an enormous problem of confidentiality.

Microfilm systems do seem to offer a good solution, however. Several copies can be made, the microfilm is easy to store and the system is quick, reliable and fairly foolproof. The viewers are cheap and even an ordinary family doctor could learn how to operate one! In one American hospital, where a few years ago notes were stored under mattresses and in closets, any patient's notes can now be found within 30 seconds, and with viewers on every ward a doctor can easily refer back to old notes. Time is saved, mistakes avoided and patients undoubtedly benefit. It is not difficult to argue that the introduction of microfilm systems would save more lives than the building of intensive care units and coronary care units. And surely saving lives and improving the quality of life is the purpose of our continuing exercise.

The reluctance of doctors to assess their techniques properly not only results in an enormous wastage of money and time, it also puts patients at risk. Ivan Illich in `Medical Nemesis; writes that `The pain, dysfunction, disability and even anguish which result from technical medical intervention now rival the morbidity due to traffic, work and even war-related activities. Only modern malnutrition is clearly ahead.'

Illich describes vividly how doctors can do harm, by reporting what has happened in Chile. In 1960, 96% of Chilean mothers breast fed their babies for over a year. By 1970, as a result of the availability of alternative, medically recommended sources of milk and the knowledge that in developed countries figure-conscious women do not breast feed, only 6% were breast feeding for a year or more and only 20% were breast feeding for two months. In other words, over 80% of breast milk is unused in Chile and the milk of 32,000 cows is needed to replace the unused natural milk. The result is that the babies and the mothers both need medical care; for the babies develop gastro-intestinal disorders and the mothers get engorged breasts. Here doctors, in true commercial spirit, have made for themselves a new nation of patients.

Illich also points out that every 24 to 36 hours between 50 per cent and 80 per cent of adults in the USA and the UK swallow a medically prescribed chemical. Since a large proportion are given or take the wrong dose or a contaminated dose, millions are poisoning themselves.

The American Food and Drug Administration estimates that one in seven of all hospital beds in the United States of America is occupied by a patient who is under treatment for toxic reactions caused by drugs given by doctors. It is estimated that the consequent financial loss amounts to 3,000 million dollars per year in the United States of America alone. It was reliably estimated in 1971 that 30,000 Americans die every year from adverse drug reactions.

According to a leading British expert, 5 per cent of the beds in general hospitals in the United Kingdom are occupied by patients suffering from the effects of treatment they have been given. A report published in the *British Medical Journal* showed that out of 1,268 patients studied, 37 had been admitted to hospital because of adverse reactions and 118 had their stay in hospital prolonged for the same reason. In all it was thought that 929 additional days of hospital care were required for this group of patients simply because of problems caused by treatment. An American survey showed that accidents are the major cause of death in young people and that accidents occur more often in hospitals than in any other place.

In a New Zealand hospital in 1972 it was reported that nearly 3 per cent of all deaths were caused by drugs. According to the WHO 'Chronicle',`.. . 1 in every 20 admissions to general hospitals is associated with an adverse reaction during treatment and 1 in every 10 hospital patients is reported to experience such a reaction while undergoing drug therapy.'

In an article entitled 'The hazards of hospitalisation' published in the *Annals of Internal Medicine*, Dr Schimmel, from the Department of Medicine at Yale University, reported on an eight-month study of 1,014 patients. He found that 198 different patients suffered 240 episodes of medically induced complications. Some reacted to drugs, others reacted to transfusions and diagnostic procedures and yet more contracted infections. In all 16 patients died from complications caused by treatment. Dr Schimmel wrote that 'each new drug and procedure bears potential hazards that are not immediately apparent and that may be discovered, like thalidomide-induced phocomelia, only after terrible harm is done', and concluded that 'the probable benefit of each test or treatment must be weighed against its possible risk.'

The most common cause of serious unwanted side effects is the administration of drugs. Often, of course, drugs can be life-saving. Patients with pneumonia would die without the use of antibiotics. But too often drugs are prescribed unnecessarily with the result that the patient is exposed to the dangers of taking a particular powerful drug without being able to take advantage of the drug's potential power to cure. Drugs that can cure serious illnesses are always powerful and powerful drugs can always cause damage. Even such useful drugs as penicillin and cortisone kill many thousands of patients. In a recent survey (published in the *British Medical Journal*) an eminent British authority, Professor Girdwood, found that in seven and a half years oral contraceptives killed 332 women, phenylbutazone killed 217 people, chlorpromazine killed 102 people, steroids killed 94 people, tranquillisers caused 257 deaths, analgesics and cough medicines caused 592 deaths and antibacterial caused 166 deaths. These figures relate only to drugs prescribed by general practitioners working in England. Even then, they probably only indicate the tip of the iceberg.

It is perhaps not surprising, therefore, that some doctors have claimed that when a patient deteriorates in hospital it should first of all be considered that he may be suffering from an adverse reaction to a drug he has been given.

Of course, it is inevitable that some patients in hospital or under treatment at home will suffer adverse effects. But it is also certain that many of the patients who suffer adverse effects need not have taken the drugs at all. A study at Johns Hopkins Hospital in Baltimore showed that hospital in-patients received an average of 15 drugs. The minimum number of drugs received by any one patient was six, the most taken was 32. It is not unreasonable to guess that a large number of those prescriptions need never have been written. After all, in one large American nursing home which had previously averaged 175 prescriptions per week, the average number of prescriptions was reduced by careful doctors to 10 a week. A survey done in 1966 in Canada in which the records of 4894 patients given antibiotics were examined showed that in 48.5 per cent of cases infection was indeed present but that in 62.5 per cent of cases the wrong drug had been prescribed. A study at the University of Arkansas Medical Centre showed that of 9,789 drug doses given by 32 nurses, there were 1,461 errors.

It is not, however, only drugs which cause problems. Medical practice has become such a sophisticated business that today even the patient going into hospital for a fairly routine operation will be subjected to numerous tests and investigations. The rarer and more complicated the condition, the more numerous the tests.

Many of the tests performed serve little purpose. For example, just about every patient going into hospital will have a routine chest X-ray. According to a recent editorial in the *British Medical Journal* these serve little or no useful purpose and are done out of tradition more than anything else. As always there is the slight but definite danger involved with any type of radiography. So here we have an example of a possibly dangerous test done for no real reason. There are many tests which are considerably more dangerous than the simple chest X-ray and which are done for no very good reason as far as the patient is concerned. Teaching hospitals, and indeed all major general hospitals, are dominated by research workers. There is a great deal of evidence to show that research is often done merely to support a career and that when the researcher is being considered for a job, no one bothers to question the purpose or usefulness of the research.

A few years ago, a medical peer wrote that 'Given some new and expensive tools such as gas chromatography, electromagnetic flowmeter or a multiple channel recorder of some kind, it becomes all too easy to find a subject for research for there is bound to be something not yet measured by this means.' The individual patient does not benefit (indeed he may suffer), society does not benefit (the research is of little use), and the only beneficiary is the researcher who, in Britain at any rate, is probably working with National Health Service resources and being paid to do some useful clinical job.

As examples of dangerous tests often done by researchers in large hospitals, I would list liver biopsy, kidney biopsy and cardiac catheterisation. Sometimes these tests provide useful results. But more often they provide nothing useful. There is, I regret to say, a mortality rate with all these procedures which are in any case often painful. At a meeting of the Royal Society of Medicine recently, it was suggested that coronary angiography is an essential investigation in all patients with angina or with chest pain of uncertain origin. A doctor from Cleveland, Ohio, has suggested that patients with a family history of heart trouble should have annual angiography. Coronary angiography is a procedure which involves taking X-rays of the heart after injecting a special substance into the heart vessels. It is a potentially dangerous procedure with a mortality rate of between 1 and 5 per cent. Similarly, it is now fairly common practice to do carotid angiography on patients with some specific symptoms. This procedure involves the taking of X-rays of the vessels supplying blood to the brain. To take the X-rays the vessels must be injected with a special dye. This again is a potentially dangerous procedure, and it is one often performed for research purposes.

As if that were not enough, in the United Kingdom in 1970 27 per cent of all known cases of food poisoning occurred in hospitals – more than in restaurants, clubs and canteens put together.

Much of the most dramatic work in hospitals goes on either in the intensive care units or in the operating theatres. I am afraid that both these two places are dangerous for the patient. Since dangerous procedures such as cardiac catheterisation and coronary angiography are common in intensive care units the patient who finds himself in one may be at much greater risk than if he had stayed at home and taken his chance there. Even operating theatres are dangerous places because of the pressures put on surgeons by hospital administrators and patients and indeed, because of their own self-imposed pressures. One eminent British transplant surgeon, writing in *The Lancet* recently, pointed out that surgeons sometimes expect to be able to do a particular operation within a certain time limit and that they may push themselves unnecessarily if they think they are falling behind time. In the USA more than 6,600 deaths occur annually as a result of mishaps with anaesthesia.

This sad catalogue of damage done by doctors and their aides is intended, not to help destroy medicine as a profession, for unlike Illich I believe that medicine has a future role, but rather to illustrate the great need for doctors to attend to the business of putting their own hospitals in order, before setting off on searches for new cures and new wonder drugs.

The damage now done by modern medical practice is enormous. In order to reduce the amount of damage, we need first of all to admit its existence, to assess its importance and to study ways of putting things right. There is more than enough work here for all the doctors and medical scientists with a yen for research. As Professor Bernard Towers, Professor of Paediatrics and Anatomy at the University of California, Los Angeles, has put it, 'It is pertinent to ask oneself whether a single case of iatrogenic disease or death, resulting directly from the careless use (misuse) of one or more of the powerful tools of modern technology, is not enough to make us pause, at least, in our current blind admiration for technological sophistication.'

Professor Towers reports that, according to conversations he has had with his former pupils, patients in London hospitals not infrequently plead with the junior doctors not to be sent, or sent back, to research units, where although they know they will be seen by the 'best brains' and given the most advanced treatment for their condition, technical procedures will be constant and unremitting. In my experience as a general practitioner this is an accurate report. Patients are becoming increasingly reluctant to enter any unit with a reputation for research.

Some of the most important contributions made by doctors to the health of their patients has involved the cessation of harmful practices. When doctors stopped bleeding their patients a century ago they saved many lives. In more recent years lives have been saved by doctors who have allowed convalescent patients to get up and who have stopped using drugs dangerously and thoughtlessly. Half a century ago bromides were recognised as dangerous and used accordingly by the more thoughtful prescribers. Twenty years ago barbiturates were found to be dangerous, as were amphetamines, but unfortunately both are still prescribed. When the doctors, mainly elderly and out of date, who still prescribe these products retire, thousands of lives will be saved.

14. Fringe Medicine

There are many fringe areas of medicine which arouse scorn among those concerned with traditional areas of medical research. There are therefore many potentially fruitful areas for curious researchers with a genuine desire to do simple research which may prove to be usefully productive.

Medicine will never be an exact science while we still do not know why the relationship between doctor and patient is so important; why it is important that the patient has faith in the doctor; why so many patients, who are given medicine by doctors they trust, do not take that medicine; why it is that different people, prescribing the same medicine, can produce different results; why a perfectly sane man with a genuine pain can obtain relief from his pain with the aid of a sugar pill, which contains absolutely nothing with any power; and so on and so on. These problems attract very little research.

Even research work is bedevilled by the inexplicable actions and reports of the people concerned. For example, researchers in one experiment told a group of intelligent subjects that they were going to conduct an experiment with two groups of rats: one group which had been trained to travel through a maze and another group which had not been so trained. The subjects then experimented with rats and proved that the rats they were told had been trained were trained. The rats that they had been told were untrained took longer to get through the maze. In fact, none of the rats was trained.

Research traditions ensure that much more research is done into finding new improved versions of existing drugs than into finding out why patients do not take the existing drugs when they are given them. Probably less than half of the patients given drugs by their doctors take them as prescribed. Some forget, some accidentally take the wrong dosage and some deliberately change their dosage schedule. It would be of far more practical use to research into why patients do not do what they are told with the powerful drugs they are given.

There is convincing evidence to show that patients with hypertension can often be controlled with placebos rather than with potentially harmful drugs, that many patients with high blood pressure are not taking their prescribed drugs properly, and that many patients with high blood pressure are not being treated properly but are being given the wrong drugs in the wrong dosages. Much of this evidence has been accumulated by accident, as a side result of work done to test new antihypertensive drugs. And yet work is still being done on new drugs, when it would seem obvious that it would be far more productive to investigate poor prescribing patterns and the unwillingness of patients to take offered advice and prescribed drugs. Surely it would be worthwhile finding out why and how hypertension can be treated without drugs?

In an article published in July 1975 in *The Lancet*, a general practitioner, working in the south of London, reported on work she had done with some of her patients with hypertension. This doctor divided a number of her patients into two groups. One group went along to the surgery regularly and spent half an hour relaxing on a couch. The other group spent the same amount of time in the surgery but were taught how to relax properly and how to meditate. The group of patients who were instructed in the art of proper relaxation and meditation made a spectacular improvement. These patients all had high blood pressure when they started their course of treatment and when they had finished most of them had quite normal blood pressures. The patients were taught over a period of three months and nine months later they were still benefiting from their learning. Since it has been known for a long time that high blood pressure is caused or aggravated by stress, the surprise is perhaps not that such a technique has been tried but that it has not been tried before! The irony is that the research was eventually done by a general practitioner without a major grant.

An editorial in *The Lancet* in May 1975 commented, 'A treatment which reduced the mean blood pressure of a group of patients from 159/100 to 139/86 mm Hg in 3 months and held it at about the same level without further medical intervention for the next 9 months would be worth a second look, provided that the baseline blood pressure had been critically assessed and a control group had been observed simultaneously. If, as a bonus, the total hypotensive drug requirements of these patients had been halved and the new treatment neither cost money nor had any side effects, it would demand very careful scrutiny. These are the results of treatment of hypertension by relaxation and meditation obtained by Patel in a South London general practice ...'.

Despite the fact that this technique costs nothing, is perfectly safe and has no side effects, there have been few other British attempts to produce similar results. The reason is, perhaps, that much medical research is done by, or sponsored on behalf of, commercial companies, and no commercial company is going to be very interested in a technique which does not involve the consumption of a marketable product. As one writer put it in a medical journal, 'Neither doctors nor patients have much truck with treatments which cannot be prescribed by pen and taken by pill.'

The South London general practitioner is not alone, however, in having produced such interesting work. In America a good many doctors have researched in this area and many have found similar results.

In material published in *Scientific American* in 1972 two American researchers, one an Assistant Professor of Medicine at Harvard Medical School, published results which showed that during transcendental meditation oxygen consumption and metabolic rates markedly decreased (more than in sleep or hypnosis) and that it is possible to measure a reduction in the level of anxiety recorded by people meditating. Physiologists in France and America have shown that some meditators can learn to slow or stop their hearts, and in April 1970 a writer in *The Lancet* showed evidence that breathing rates per minute drop significantly during transcendental meditation. Researchers at the University of Cologne showed that meditators have reduced levels of aggression, depression, irritability and nervousness and researchers at Stanford Research Institute have shown that those who learn meditation manage without, or with smaller doses of psychotropic drugs.

Subjects have learned to control their own heart rate, blood pressure and the electrical activity of the brain. It is possible to learn to control muscle tension and so to relieve headaches, backache and so on. Researchers, first intrigued by the fact that monks or yogis who achieve self-control during transcendental meditation can slow their heart rate to such an extent that little blood is being pumped around and no heartbeat can be heard, can sweat on command and can even draw air or water into the intestines through the anus, have trained perfectly ordinary people to do similar things. Electrodes are attached to the body and connected to a pulse meter which enables the subject to see or hear his heart rate. The subject then imagines situations which affect his heart rate, either making it beat faster or slower. Eventually the subject learns to control his heart rate without the pulse meter. It is not a difficult exercise.

There are a great number of conditions which experts believe can eventually be controlled without outside help. I have explained how patients can learn how to control their blood pressure and their heart rate. In similar ways, patients can learn how to control their appetite by controlling the compulsion to eat. Volunteers have learned how to control their own skin temperature, either increasing or reducing the flow of blood into the blood vessels. Such controls could help patients with recurrent headaches and with poor circulation. It has been suggested, by workers in Kansas, that tumours could be starved of blood.

People with muscle tension or muscle fatigue can also benefit by learning how to relax their muscles. Patients with excessive acid secretion can learn to control the flow of acid and, hence, the formation of peptic ulcers, and patients with respiratory disorders can also learn to control their own lungs.

It is not, of course, possible for any patient to improve the efficiency of a deteriorating organ where that organ has suffered an irreversible change. If, for example, the heart has a large chunk of dead muscle, there is nothing the owner can do to 'cure' that. Biofeedback, as it is called, can, however, help to cure temporary problems (such as irregular beating) and to prevent the development of disorders exacerbated by stress. Very little research work has been done in this area; and yet the possibilities are tremendous and the costs minimal.

There are many other fringe areas of medicine which merit investigation. An obvious subject for thorough study is acupuncture. Despite the fact that this is one of the oldest forms of medical treatment, there is very little scientific literature on the subject. Few proper trials have been done and mention of the subject in many medical centres is likely to bring only laughter and scorn. The attitude of doctors in this instance, is similar to that of the native who cannot understand a piece of equipment. He is frightened of it and to conceal his fear he laughs.

Acupuncture is said to have developed after soldiers wounded in battle thousands of years ago noticed that they sometimes recovered from long-lasting illnesses after being wounded by arrows. There are 900 acupuncture sites and traditionally the needles are made of silver. There has been a great argument within society about acupuncture for many ears. Sir William Osler once wrote that 'For lumbago, acupuncture is, in acute cases, the most efficient treatment'. Aldous Huxley summed up our attitude to acupuncture by saying `... that a needle stuck into one's foot should improve the functioning of one's liver is obviously incredible. The only trouble is that, as a matter of empirical fact, it does happen.'

A number of doctors have made subjective trials of acupuncture and been impressed. In February 1972 Professor J.P. Payne, Professor of Anaesthetics at the Royal College of Surgeons, wrote, 'Despite the scepticism of doctors trained in Western methods there is now enough corroborative evidence to suggest that acupuncture is sufficiently successful in relieving pain to warrant detailed investigation'.

In 1970 a total of 400,000 cases of acupuncture anaesthesia were reported in the People's Republic of China, the advantages being a lack of side effects, the speed of recovery from the operation, the cheapness of the technique and the fact that no expensive equipment is needed. In January 1974 four American surgeons wrote in *American Surgeon* that they had treated over 300 patients in and around the New York area by acupuncture. The surgeons wrote that, in over three quarters of the cases, they found that acupuncture is one of the most effective treatments for arthritis, neuralgia and skeletomuscular pain. Two doctors writing in the *Canadian Anaesthetists Society Journal* in 1974 wrote that 'Reports of a large number of surgical cases operated under acupuncture anaesthesia with a success rate of up to 90 per cent have now sufficiently substantiated that the effectiveness of acupuncture can no longer be doubted and that it has to be examined seriously.' DeBakey, the heart surgeon, is quoted as having said that 'We should continue to examine it until we do have a rational explanation that either confirms or denies its usefulness.'

One author writing in the *Medical Journal of Australia* in January 1974 suggested that the stimulation from the needles disrupts or overrides the stimuli coming from other parts of the body and that as a consequence the brain loses its normal picture of the body as a whole. Meanwhile, it seems to me illogical to dismiss out of hand, a safe and apparently effective treatment and yet to accept, happily, dangerous and only equally effective drug treatments. It is useless to argue that acupuncture uses a type of hypnosis and to dismiss the technique for that reason. If it is a type of hypnosis, it is surely still worthy of scientific study.

There are many other para-medical treatments and theories which merit close investigation but which, because they run outside the usual stream of discoveries, and because they do not fit neatly into the medical profession's idea of how things should be tackled have been ignored. Denis Burkitt, for example, has gained relatively little recognition from the medical profession for his theory that if we all ate more fibre we would suffer from fewer large bowel disorders. He bases his theory on the observation that many bowel disorders (such as diverticulitis and ulcerative colitis) are rare in Africa though Africans get them when they eat a Western diet. He says that bowel diseases have been on the increase since white flour was introduced in 1885.

Another nutritional theory is that put forward by Roger MacDougall, a man who claims to have cured himself of multiple sclerosis by putting himself on a special diet. MacDougall argues that doctors are taught that nerve tissues cannot be repaired when damaged, but his theory is that since multiple sclerosis is a condition caused by the degeneration of the myelin sheath surrounding nerves and since the only known treatment for a degenerative disease is a gluten-free diet, it makes sense to him to follow a gluten-free diet. He cannot offer evidence for his theory but offers cured followers instead. One of them, a biochemist, wrote a letter to *The Lancet* supporting the theory, but few researchers have seemed interested enough to tackle such a controversial cure: to either prove it or disprove it.

The feeling that too many medical researchers are working in areas where the potential benefit does not equal the necessary expenditure of effort is growing. As Professor Alan H. Williams of the Department of Economics at the University of York said at a recent Royal Society of Medicine Symposium, `I do not see a great deal of effort devoted to designing better chairs for arthritic old women and matters of that kind. Such things may be far more important to the welfare of the community than some of the things we read about in the scientific journals'. Much research is done on basic problems and can be classed as 'gambling' rather than research. Many disease processes have their origins in our surroundings but researchers have for half a century focused their interest on disorders of function and structure.

According to an editorial in the magazine `General Practitioner' on 22 September 1975, even the British Health Minister, Dr David Owen ` ... believes that the Medical Research Council spends too much on esoteric projects and insufficient on widespread complaints which account for millions of lost working days a year – not to mention untold suffering'. The editorial writer also pointed out that more than half of all the time taken off work by dockers, miners and many other workers in heavy industries is due to back trouble, that back pain costs about £200 million a year in Britain, that on any day 50,000 men and women are off work with back pain, that 1½ million people visit their doctors in the course of a year complaining of backache, and that the amount allocated by the Department of Health and Social Security for research into back pain during 1975/6 is a miserly £75,000. Judging by the cost of the average research project these days, that should just about pay for an office boy, a filing cabinet and an office cat.

Other subjects receiving comparatively little attention include the facts that cold weather helps to cause heart attacks, and that carbon disulphide may also cause heart attacks. Less than 0.01 per cent of NHS expenditure is spent on health education. In under-developed countries we still more or less ignore the problem of overpopulation. The human reproductory apparatus was designed to make it possible for a man and a woman to have ten or more children, so that one or two would survive. However, as health care improves, this reproductory capacity becomes more and more of an embarrassment. We lower the child mortality rate in developing countries by clearing up some of the infections of infancy, but then, because of malnutrition, the children we save die a more horrible death a few years later.

Just as surely as there are areas of medicine where further research is not needed at the present time, so are there areas where research is desperately needed. I hope that these last three chapters have helped to describe convincingly some of the gaps in our knowledge.

15. The Final Assessment

Medical research, and indeed the practice of medicine itself, can at present be divided into three broad categories. First, there is the traditional type of medical practice, as exemplified by the general practitioner on his home visits and in his surgery, looking after the acute and chronic sick. This type of medicine is basically therapeutic, in so far as the doctor is mainly concerned with keeping his patients alive and well and restoring them to health when they fall ill. General practice relies more on the personal relationship between doctor and patient than on medical technology. This type of medical care is fairly costly, but it is the most important branch of medicine as far as most patients are concerned. The current expenditure on research in this area is minimal.

Second, there is the type of medical research and practice which aims at providing temporary solutions to individual problems, usually in a hospital or clinic. This type of technology is well illustrated by the artificial dialysis machine and the heart transplant. These are expensive research projects. They are only marginally effective and provide a technical support for the doctor involved in general practice.

The third, and probably most productive, type of medicine is that which helps to improve the quality and quantity of life for people as a whole rather than for individuals. This branch of medicine and research includes the use of, and search for, vaccination materials, the provision of health education programmes and the provision of effective screening programmes, as well as the design and management of public health measures.

Most of the money which is available for health care and for medical research is spent on programmes which fall into the second category. The health services in the developed countries are geared to the care of those with rare and medically interesting diseases, and the research programmes naturally aim at providing the existing health services with supplies of information. Those who suffer from such unusual and uncommon disorders as haemophilia and porphyria receive priority, while the aged, the worn out, the chronically sick, the psychologically ill, the uninteresting, the useless, the unfashionably ill, and the working man in an unhealthy environment, all receive little or no attention. The Director General of the World Health Organisation complained in the August/September (1975) issue of the magazine *World Health* that 'Vast technological resources are deployed to cope with the small number of sophisticated diseases while the prevention of disease and promotion of health definitely take second place.'

There are a number of reasons why money is spent on research into methods of dealing with incurable disorders. The first is that, traditionally, doctors have always believed that a greater understanding of the disease processes will lead to an increased ability to cope with them. There is not, however, very much evidence to show that our research programmes over the last century or so have contributed much to the actual practice of medicine or had any real effort on mortality or morbidity rates.

Through the expenditure of a great deal of money and effort we have learned much about the basic physiology of the human body. That knowledge, however, is still of little real value. We know that a cell contains a nucleus and we know the secrets of DNA, but that information does not help the doctor visiting a man with bronchitis or a heart attack. We know a great deal about the functioning of the liver but we still do not really know why an aspirin tablet works. We know much about infectious diseases, but we still cannot deal with the common cold.

The second reason why we spend so much money and effort on research intended to find treatments for existing diseases is that medical researchers tend to base their work on the fact that medical practice involves a one-to-one relationship between doctor and patient. The doctor treats the patient and is paid by him, or his representatives, for the care he provides. Doctors, and hence researchers, are more interested in treating a sick person than in keeping a healthy one healthy.

One other reason for our spending money on patients who are ill, rather than on people who are not yet ill, is that the man who has a chronic heart disease is real. When we are talking about candidates for open heart surgery (or kidney transplantation or whatever) we are talking about real, identifiable people. It is possible to go into a hospital and sit by the bed of a man who will benefit from an open heart operation. It is possible to see him recover for a while after the operation and to see him live on for a year or two longer.

On the other hand, the people who will benefit from campaigns to stop smoking, or cut down the amount of pollution in the atmosphere, do not seem real. We do not know who these faceless people are. You cannot go into a hospital and see the man who does not have bronchitis or who does not have lung cancer. And yet the men with chronic bronchitis and the men who will be saved from chronic bronchitis, are just as real as the men with real heart disease. Each one of them has a family, friends, a job, a hobby and probably a mortgage. The point is that for the cost of a single open heart operation, we can probably save a dozen men from getting chronic bronchitis.

On humanitarian grounds, therefore, it would be reasonable to spend more money on preventive medicine and less on curative medicine and research. It can also be argued that there are economic advantages to be obtained from spending money on preventive medicine.

Consider again our man with chronic bronchitis who develops the disease in his late forties, who is disabled at the age of 55 and who dies at the age of 65. It will cost several thousand pounds to provide this man with medical care and to make social security payments to him and his family. The nation will lose his potential productivity when he is not at work. He will have become a burden on society.

It is not difficult to explain why, on economic, social and humanitarian grounds, it is better to spend money on preventive medicine than on almost any aspect of medical research or high-powered hospital medicine. We have, over the last few years, spent hundreds of millions of pounds on searching for a cure for cancer. If we had spent that same amount of money on preventive medicine, designed to cut down the incidence of cancer, there is no doubt at all that a large number – probably half – of the people with cancer today would not have cancer. All we have to do is to protect ourselves against those chemicals that induce perhaps 80 per cent of cancers. We have also spent many millions of pounds over the last few years on searching for better ways to treat the man with a coronary; yet when it comes to the crunch the two most important weapons we have are digitalis and morphia – both drugs which have been available for centuries. If we had spent our money on persuading healthy people to stop smoking, lose weight, take more exercise and so on, we would have cut down the number of people having heart attacks by half. We have spent millions on looking after the victims of road accidents, with only moderate success. If we had spent just a small amount of that money on preventing accidents, on ensuring that cars, roadside furniture and drivers were better designed and prepared for battle, the number of people injured and killed would have been greatly reduced. The man saved from injury is just as real as the injured man who is saved.

Of course, I am not suggesting that we spend all our money on preventive medicine and none at all on research. There are, as I have already described, many areas where more research is needed. What I am suggesting is that we look more critically at medical research and decide just where we want to spend our limited amounts of money.

We none of us like to admit that choices like this have to be made. We try to hide from them and let other people take the decisions. The result is that we spend our money on what the doctors and researchers want to spend it on. Each country has only a limited amount of money to spend on medicine and has to decide whether the best results will be obtained by spending that money on curative medicine, or on preventive medicine. They must also decide just how much they want to spend on research.

Researchers themselves, of course, always object when it is suggested that they should be told what to do. They like the freedom they enjoy at present, the freedom of being able to do what they want. Doctors, in general, encourage the spending of money on research into methods of treatment, since only by so doing will the demand for medical skills increase. The researchers who object to doing work on commission argue that they need to be treated like artists, that they need to have freedom. In so arguing, they forget that many masterpieces of art were commissioned and finished for cash.

Society provides the funds and other resources for research, and it is quite entitled to specify the general directions in which that research should move. In doing so, we will do well to remember that work directed towards the improvement of human health will inevitably add to our store of information, while work designed to add to that store will not necessarily improve the quality and quantity of life.

Further Reading

Rather than merely including here long, forbidding lists of books and journals consulted during the preparation of this book, I have put references in the text where I think they are needed. In addition I have here compiled a short list of books which I feel might be of particular interest to those who wish to continue their study of the subject.

Beecher, H.K. Research and the individual: Human Studies, Little, Brown, Boston (USA) 1970

Burnet, F.M., Genes, Dreams and Realities, Medical and Technical Publishing Co., Lancaster 1971

Clark, M., Medicine Today: A report on a decade of progress, Funk (USA) 1960

Cochrane, A.L., Effectiveness and Efficiency, Nuffield Provincial Hospitals Trust 1972

Coleman, V.E, The Medicine Men, Temple Smith 1975

Cooper, M., Rationing Health Care, Croom Helm 1975

Delgado, J.M.R., Physical Control of the Mind, Harper & Row, New York 1969

Dixon,B., What is Science For?, Collins 1973

Dorozynski, A., Doctors and Healers, International Development Research Centre 1975

Fox, R.C., Experiment Perilous, Free Press (USA) 1959

Fehr R. and Kunz R. (Eds), 'The challenge of life, Roche Anniversary Symposium, International Publications Service, Basle 1971

Glaser, H. The Drama of Medicine, Lutterworth 1962

Glemser B., Man Against Cancer: Research and Progress, Bodley Head 1969

Greenberg, S., The quality of mercy: a report on the critical condition of hospitals and medical care in the USA, Atheneum, New York 1971

Illich, I., Medical Nemesis, Calder & Boyers 1974

Illingworth, C., The Sanguine Mystery, Nuffield Provincial Hospitals Trust 1970

Klein, G. and Haddow, A., Advances in Cancer Research (annual publication); Academy Press

Koestler, A., The Roots of Coincidence, Hutchinson 1972

Lang, R.W., The Politics of Drugs, Saxon House 1974

McLachlan, G. (Ed.), Problems and Progress in Medical Care, Nuffield Provincial Hospitals Trust 1972

Patient, Doctor, Society, Nuffield Provincial Hospitals Trust 1972

McLachlan, G. and McKeown, T. (Eds), Medical History and Medical Care, Nuffield Provincial Hospitals Trust 1971

McKeown, T. and Lowe, O.R., An Introduction to Social Medicine,

Blackwell, Oxford 1966

Miller, H., Medicine and Society, OUP 1973

Neal, H.E., Disease Detectives: your career in medical research, Messner, New York 1968

Newell, K.W. (Ed.), Health by the People, WHO 1975

Powell,J.E., A New Look at Medicine and Politics, Pitman Medical 1966

Rachman, J. and Philips, C., Psychology and Medicine, Temple Smith 1974

Robin, A. and Macdonald, D., Lessons in Leucotomy, Kimpton 1975

Rorvik, D., As Man Becomes Machine, Souvenir Press 1973

Selye, H., From Dream to Discovery: on Being a Scientist, McGraw-Hill, New York 1964

Stevens, R., American Medicine and the Public Interest, Yale 1974

Titmuss, R.M., The Gift of Relationship, Allen & Unwin 1970

Wolstenholme, G.E.W. and O'Connor, M. (Eds), 'Ethics in Medical Progress: with special reference to transplantation, Churchill 1966

In addition, the following HMSO publications may be of interest: Annual Report on Departmental Research and Development from the Department of Health and Social Security (1973/4) Report of the Working Party on the Experimental Manipulation of the Genetic Composition of Micro-organisms (1975) Cancer Research 1972, A Framework for Government Research and Development (White Paper) 1972

Printed in Great Britain
by Amazon

20577075R10098